Supporting Children's Mental Health and Wellbeing

Supporting Children's Mental Health and Wellbeing

A Strength-Based Approach for Early Childhood Educators

Jean Barbre, EdD, LMFT
and Ingrid Anderson, EdD

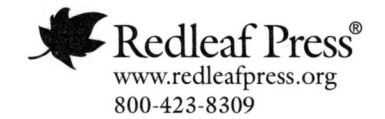

Redleaf Press®
www.redleafpress.org
800-423-8309

Published by Redleaf Press
10 Yorkton Court
St. Paul, MN 55117
www.redleafpress.org

© 2022 by Jean Barbre and Ingrid Anderson

All rights reserved. Unless otherwise noted on a specific page, no portion of this publication may be reproduced or transmitted in any form or by any means, electronic or mechanical, including photocopying, recording, or capturing on any information storage and retrieval system, without permission in writing from the publisher, except by a reviewer, who may quote brief passages in a critical article or review to be printed in a magazine or newspaper, or electronically transmitted on radio, television, or the internet.

First edition 2021
Cover design by Cathy Challman
Cover photograph by iStock/FatCamera
Interior design by Becky Daum
Typeset in Adobe Garamond Pro
Printed in the United States of America
29 28 27 26 25 24 23 22   1 2 3 4 5 6 7 8

Library of Congress Cataloging-in-Publication Data

Names: Barbre, Jean, author. | Anderson, Ingrid Mari, 1967- author.
Title: Supporting children's mental health and wellbeing : a strength-based approach for early childhood educators / by Jean Barbre and Ingrid Anderson.
Description: First edition. | St. Paul, MN : Redleaf Press, 2021. | Includes bibliographical references and index. | Summary: "The emotional lives of young children are growing increasingly more complex. This book incorporates strength-based child care strategies to foster positive reciprocal relationships between caregiver and young children and strengthen children's resiliency and wellbeing"— Provided by publisher.
Identifiers: LCCN 2021038794 (print) | LCCN 2021038795 (ebook) | ISBN 9781605547428 (paperback) | ISBN 9781605547435 (ebook)
Subjects: LCSH: Mentally ill children--Care. | Children--Family relationships. | Well-being.
Classification: LCC RJ499.B32 2021 (print) | LCC RJ499 (ebook) | DDC 362.2083--dc23
LC record available at https://lccn.loc.gov/2021038794
LC ebook record available at https://lccn.loc.gov/2021038795

Printed on acid-free paper

To Mom, who led by example of what it means to champion and advocate for young children. I love you.
—Ingrid

To Carly, Charlie, and Sam. May you live happy, healthy, and extraordinary lives.
—Jean

"Instead of raising children who turn out okay despite their childhood, let's raise children who turn out extraordinary because of their childhood."
—L. R. Knost, *Two Thousand Kisses a Day: Gentle Parenting through the Ages and Stages*

CONTENTS

Acknowledgments ix

Section 1: The Circle of Caregiver and Child Wellbeing 1

Chapter 1: The Foundations of Mental Health and Wellness — 7
Chapter 2: Mental Health and Wellbeing — 25
Chapter 3: Caregiver Wellbeing — 34
Chapter 4: The Six Pillars of Strength-Based Caregiving — 48

Section 2: The Six Pillars 61

Chapter 5: Pillar One: Social and Emotional Development — 62
Chapter 6: Pillar Two: Attachment and Caregiving Relationships — 82
Chapter 7: Pillar Three: Understanding Concerning Behaviors — 97
Chapter 8: Pillar Four: Risk and Resiliency — 107
Chapter 9: Pillar Five: Family Relationships and Culture — 124
Chapter 10: Pillar Six: Caregiver's Sphere of Influence — 139

Section 3: Strength-Based Classroom Strategies 149

Chapter 11: Strength-Based Classroom Approaches and Resources — 150
Chapter 12: Becoming a Strength-Based Caregiver — 172

Appendix A: Recommended Children's Books for Social and Emotional Development 177

Appendix B: Websites and Internet Resources 179

References 181

Index 185

Acknowledgments

Writing a book is like embarking on a long adventure. You set off on your journey, never sure of what you might encounter. We would like to thank our guides, who along the way offered sage advice, reflected with a kind yet critical eye, and encouraged us to continue along the path until we arrived.

We'd like to thank the wonderful staff at Redleaf Press, including Melissa York, Renee Hammes, Douglas Schmitz, and Meredith Burks, for enthusiastically supporting our desire to write *Supporting Children's Mental Health and Wellbeing: A Strength-Based Approach for Early Childhood Educators*. You have made this book a pleasure to work on. We appreciate the opportunity to share our knowledge and expertise on early mental health and wellbeing with the caregivers who care for young children every day.

We'd like to thank Kathryn Buechel, PhD, for her advice on the strength-based holistic activities and yoga exercises. We would also like to thank our colleagues in the Infant/Toddler Mental Health program at Portland State University for their support and understanding of infant and toddler mental health that started us on this journey.

We want to thank the countless early childhood educators we have worked with throughout our careers who have shown us what it means to advocate for and promote the mental health and wellbeing of our youngest learners. Thank you all for your compassion and daily commitment to helping all children learn, grow, and thrive.

We'd like to thank our family, friends, and colleagues for their interest and encouragement as we wrote this book—in particular, our spouses, Greg and Brett, who saw more of our computer screens than our faces during this time. We deeply appreciate your patience and understanding through the many adventures we have navigated over the past several decades.

SECTION 1

The Circle of Caregiver and Child Wellbeing

During the first five years of life, young children are busy exploring and learning about the world. They are developing skills across all five developmental domains: cognitive, linguistical, physical, and especially social and emotional. We believe that adult-child relationships and social and emotional skills are foundational to a child's mental health and wellbeing. Early attachments to loving, caring adults help children develop feelings of security and trust, providing them with the skills they need to form close relationships with others, adapt to the changing situations of life, and develop a sense of self and wellbeing.

We wrote *Supporting Children's Mental Health and Wellbeing: A Strength-Based Approach for Early Childhood Educators* to support early child care providers as they navigate the changing emotional climate of the children and families in their care. This book is designed to help those who work in early care and education understand the relationship between mental health and typical social and emotional development. We hope that by reading this book, you will gain a deeper understanding of the early mental health and wellbeing of children ages birth through five and learn strength-based, developmentally appropriate strategies you can use to support young children's social and emotional development.

A Strength-Based Approach

Strength-based caregiving is the ability to reflect on which practices best support each child's individual needs. When we incorporate a strength-based approach, we start with what is present—skills and competencies that already exist within the child and family. In this approach, focus is placed on the child's and family's positive attributes rather than on their deficits. A deficit-based approach sees what is lacking rather than what is present. We want to ask ourselves, *How do I build on* _____? rather than, *Why can't they* _____? When we use a strength-based approach and language, we orient ourselves to working with families. A strength-based approach recognizes individual, family, and environmental strengths. We see the strength of the individual child and their unique capabilities. We acknowledge the strength that comes from their environments, including cultural identity. We build on family strengths by recognizing their resourcefulness and resiliency.

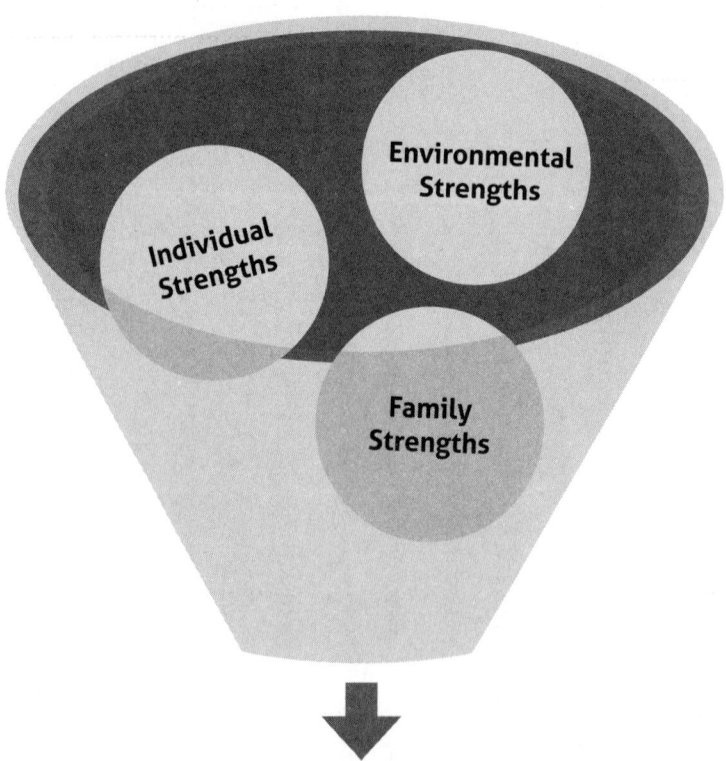

Strength-Based Approaches

For caregivers, the foundation of strength-based caregiving is the dyadic or one-child/one-adult relationship. The dyadic relationship is fundamentally different from our relationship with a group or classroom of children. A dyadic relationship is mutually engaging. For example, an infant and their primary caregiver engage in serve and return, or behaviors in which each individual in the pair reads facial and body expressions and responds to the other in a back-and-forth pattern. Dyadic relationships are a cornerstone of healthy attachment, brain development, and social and emotional development.

The dyadic relationship requires trust and respect between both members of the dyad. In this relationship, the caregiver trusts that the child's behavior is genuine and the child trusts the caregiver to meet their needs. As caregivers, we need to recognize that misbehavior emerges from underlying unmet needs. As parent educator Dr. Jane Nelsen states, "Misbehaving children are discouraged children who have mistaken ideas on how to achieve their primary goal—to belong" (Nelsen 2021). All children have a profound need to feel human connections and a sense of belonging. They need their hopes for the future to be nurtured. Each individual child needs their caregivers to treat them with respect and attribute positive intention to their actions.

A strength-based approach requires caregivers to build a culture of trust and respect with each child and their family. Building mutually respectful relationships begins with our first encounters with young children and their families as we create space to build trust with families and enter a relationship that sees every child's limitless potential. Building on a child's strengths invites families to feel safe in having complex, and sometimes courageous, conversations about their children. Families will understand that we see the whole child, not just the child's challenges.

Why We Wrote This Book

We the authors each come from unique backgrounds that frame our understanding of child mental health and wellbeing. We each have over thirty years of experience working in early childhood programs and mental health, and hold doctoral degrees in education.

Jean is a licensed marriage and family therapist, early childhood administrator, and university faculty member. She has extensive advanced training as a certified trauma therapist and in holistic supports for young children in mindfulness and yoga practices.

Ingrid has been an early childhood educator and administrator, and is now a faculty member in graduate programs for infant and toddler mental health and inclusive early childhood education. She has an advanced degree in conflict resolution and peaceable solutions skills. Her work has focused on access and equity issues in early childhood, and her research focuses on the wellbeing of early childhood educators and young children.

We both have trained as parent educators and have worked together since 1998. In our collaborations, we have established and managed preschool programs, collaborated with local mental health supports, and taught and researched at various universities around the world. Over the past two decades, we have seen the early care and education field face increasingly more complex challenges in scaffolding social and emotional development. As we worked, presented, and collaborated together, we began noticing requests for guidance supports from the early childhood field increasing. Caregivers were expressing concerns that the strategies they were using to guide young children were not as effective as in the past.

Concurrently, we have seen a growing interest among early child care providers to understand early mental health and wellbeing. There are now more advances in mental health and empirical evidence about developmental disorders available for mental health professionals than ever before, but we know that this information is not readily available to early childhood providers. In 2016 early childhood advocacy group Zero to Three released the *Diagnostic Classification of Mental Health and Developmental Disorders of Infancy and Early Childhood DC:0–5* (Zero to Three 2016). This document provides general diagnostic information for mental health clinicians but is not written for the early child care provider. Therefore, we decided to write this book to help caregivers understand the continuum leading from social and emotional development to mental health and wellbeing.

Our goal is to equip caregivers with the tools they need to address children's development based on mutual respectful dyadic relationships in the classroom. We want to help caregivers build their practices on a strength-based approach with the resources they need to thrive alongside the children in their care. This book represents a culmination of our work together in thinking about early childhood educators, young children, their families, and the changing social and emotional landscapes of the early childhood classroom.

We will provide an overview of major mental health disorders commonly seen in early childhood environments. Our intention is to educate and inform early childhood providers in understanding mental health and wellbeing in young children. This book is in *no way* meant for you to label or diagnose children with a mental health disorder. The information in this book *is not* a substitute for the knowledge, skill, and expertise of qualified mental health professionals. Should you have any health, medical,

SECTION 1

or disability questions or concerns about the children in your care, please follow your agency's protocol for referrals to a licensed physician or other health care professional.

> As we examine supporting children's mental health and wellbeing, we must first identify the common terms and definitions used in this book. They are as follows.
>
> - **Mental Health:** The sense of wellbeing an individual possesses that impacts how they think and feel about, adapt to, and cope with the stresses of life.
> - **Mental Illness:** A wide range of conditions and disorders that affect an individual's behavior, mood, and thinking. A mental health professional must diagnose a mental disorder, which meets specific criteria using a common diagnostic tool. See more information on diagnostic tools in chapter 2.
> - **Wellbeing**: A positive sense of self that allows individuals to lead happy, productive lives and form and maintain healthy relationships.
> - **Emotional Wellbeing:** The quality of emotional responses to life experiences, including the ability to adapt and change, demonstrate resiliency, resolve conflict, manage emotions, and generate consistent feelings of happiness and hopefulness.
> - **Social Health**: The skills and competencies needed to form healthy relationships and social interactions. These include skills and competencies to communicate with others, work cooperatively in groups, have our needs met, and form relationships.
> - **Emotional Health**: The ability at a developmentally appropriate age level to develop, understand, express, and navigate a wide range of human emotions.
>
> Mental health and wellbeing are used interchangeably in this book, and the concepts apply to both adults and children. Social and emotional health specifically refers to children's skills and competencies within that developmental domain. More information on social and emotional development is found in chapter 5.

We congratulate you for exploring the mental health and wellbeing of young children. Sometimes this exploration reminds us of our own journeys and the relationships and events that have influenced who we are as adults, so we have provided numerous practices in this book to help you reflect on your own understanding of mental health. We know that the adult's emotional health influences the child's emotional health, so we hope that these reflective practices will provide you opportunities to foster your own personal growth to allow you to better serve the children in your care. Enjoy the journey! We believe that the more you learn about yourself and grow as a person, the more caring and compassionate you will be as a professional early care provider.

CHAPTER 1

The Foundations of Mental Health and Wellness

Every day in a hundred small ways our children ask, "Do you see me? Do you hear me? Do I matter?" Their behaviour often reflects our response.
—L. R. Knost, A Gentle Parent

Mental health, which includes social and emotional development, affects how we think, feel, and respond to the people and situations around us. Historically, clinical knowledge, therapeutic models, and interventions surrounding mental health and mental disorders have been available for adults, adolescents, and older children but have lagged for younger children, especially children ages birth though five. In 2020 researchers found that one in six children between the ages of two and eight suffers from one or more mental, behavioral, or developmental disorders (Centers for Disease Control and Prevention 2020c). Disorders such as autism spectrum disorder, attention deficit hyperactivity disorder, sensory processing disorders, anxiety disorders, and mood disorders, or combinations of several such disorders can be diagnosed in young children.

We know that a significant number of children and families experience complex life circumstances that present serious challenges for developing children. A child's mental health and wellbeing can be affected by family structures, home and community living conditions, diagnosed disabilities, and trauma, to name a few factors. Solutions for supporting young children are not always simple because disorders surface from complicated, ongoing familial or systemic socioeconomic living conditions. Therefore, strength-based supports need to be individualized, focusing on the ongoing needs of each child.

Young children are rapidly growing and changing, and their responses to emotional experiences and traumatic events differ from those of older children and adults. We know that early disruptions in the developmental process of young children can potentially leave a lasting impact on a child's capacity to learn, make decisions, and form future relationships. Whether it is a single traumatic event or a recurring situation, all traumatic experiences impact developing children. This heartbreaking information means it is critical that those who provide care for young children acquire a deeper understanding of early mental health and what they can do to provide optimal care. The impact of trauma on the developing child is further discussed in chapter 8.

Actions such as aggression, tantrums, and noncompliance have new meaning when the underlying needs of the young child are identified and addressed. When confronted with complex behaviors and concerns for the wellbeing of a child and their classmates, we ask ourselves the following questions:

- How do I handle children's complex social and emotional development?
- How do I get to the underlying causes of children's strong emotions?
- What supports are available to me to manage children's complex behaviors?
- How can I partner with families to support their children?
- How can I access resources to meet the needs of the child and the family?
- How do I prevent myself from experiencing burnout in my caregiving job?

This book is designed to answer these questions and many more. We explore the importance of creating high-quality and strength-based environments where relationships are central to the child's growing sense of self and wellbeing. In particular, we focus on the dyadic relationship, or the one-to-one relationship between a primary caregiver and a developing child, because we know that the child's first and most important relationship is with the adult who provides their primary care. Relationships with caring adults are foundational in helping a child develop their sense of self and wellbeing. Understanding early mental health is key to equipping children with the healthy social and emotional skills they need to lead happy and productive lives.

This chapter presents an overview of the components influencing the whole child's growth and development. In reflecting on children's development, we begin with understanding the role of family and community. Next, we address the role of responsive caregiving and the importance of loving and nurturing care to young children's growth and development. We know that children's brains are strongly influenced by their experiences and the care they receive. Early brain functioning influences children's behavior and sense of wellbeing throughout their lifetime. High-quality learning environments provide optimal care and development while guiding the formation of young children's relationships. Because children learn through play, environments that provide multiple opportunities to engage in play are a foundation of children's learning. These components provide the landscape of social and emotional wellbeing, and it begins with families and communities.

Families and Communities

We know that family and communities greatly influence how a child develops and learns to respond to life's situations and events. Beginning at birth, children learn who they are in the world and how to interact and communicate with those around them. The world young children are growing up in today is dramatically different from that of any previous generation. Today's children live in a rapidly changing culture greatly influenced by advances in technology and the internet. Nearly thirty years ago, the early childhood field entered a period of rapid growth that has yet to slow down. Today the majority of parents work outside the home, and children ages birth through five are spending more and more time in the care of others in various settings, including child care centers, family child care facilities, or the homes of family, friends, or neighbors. Regardless of the setting, all children deserve nurturing and responsive care provided by knowledgeable and well-trained care providers. As the field of child care evolves and changes, we see a continued focus on children's social and emotional development and how adults, including early care providers, can support children's sense of wellbeing. As caregivers, we need to reflect on how we nurture children as critical thinkers, collaborators, communicators, and creators/innovators. These skills, which are part of responsive caregiving, emerge from children's social and emotional mental health and last a lifetime.

Responsive Caregiving

Early childhood caregivers who spend a majority of days with the child are considered primary caregivers. As such, you partner with other primary caregivers in young children's lives based on the makeup of the family unit. Family units can include any combination of one parent, both parents, family members like grandparents, or other designated legal guardians. Primary care includes providing food, shelter, comfort, cognitive stimulation, and emotional support by feeding, changing diapers, rocking, soothing, talking, interacting, and engaging. For the purpose of this book, the terms *caregiver* and *primary caregiver* will be used interchangeably with you, the reader. Regardless of who this person is, their role in the adult-child dyad is paramount to establishing the child's foundation of mental health and wellbeing.

Responsive caregiving fosters healthy social and emotional development, as caring adults accurately interpret children's cues and meet their ongoing needs. Brain research shows that contrary to the historical practice of letting children fuss and cry, adults build trust by appropriately responding to young children's needs. Since young children are so dependent on adults to meet all their needs, their foundation of wellbeing begins with trust built through the development of respectful reciprocal relationships. These secure relationships provide children with feelings of love, trust, and security. In secure relationships, caregivers are responsive to the children's ongoing needs. Like secure relationships, attachment also allows children to feel protected, comforted, and loved.

Beginning in infancy, attachment develops between the young child and one or two specific stable adults, typically parents or another primary adult in the child's life. Attachment is more complex and profound than a secure relationship. We learn to love, care for, and form close, intimate relationships with others from the people who first cared for us. Nurturing, responsive caregivers help children feel safe, loved, and secure during these formative years. Therefore, infants, toddlers, and preschool children begin learning to love and care for others during their first relationships with adults. These early experiences and relationships influence the developing brain and form the beginnings of children's mental health and wellbeing.

The Developing Brain

We know the brain is wired for relationships. Because children are rapidly growing and changing, it is important to examine how relationships influence the developing brain. The human brain is a dynamic organ that changes and adapts throughout one's lifetime. In the early years, a child's brain is establishing important neurological pathways; therefore, positive nurturing environments that promote social and emotional development are critical during this period. During the first five years, the brain is more flexible than at any other time, setting the stage for a lifetime of learning. This period of growth, called neuroplasticity, allows the developing brain to change and adapt with alarming speed.

The developing brain is profoundly influenced by the presence or absence of experiences, including loving and nurturing care. For example, when caregivers respond warmly and caringly to a young child's cries, the child's brain makes a positive connection to the adult's nurturing response and the surrounding environment. Through both attachment to caregivers and the quality of care they receive, young children strengthen positive brain connections that promote wellbeing. They develop internal connections or feelings that the environment and the adults around them will meet their needs and bring them comfort. These feelings are internalized and hardwired as safety, security, and trust, which are foundational to creating a state of wellbeing. These neurological pathways affect the ways we think, learn, and manage emotions. Early brain connections affect how we build relationships with others, show empathy, care for others, and demonstrate compassion. We know that the neurological pathways formed in the early years and the quality of care received influences a person for their lifetime. Therefore, early nurturing, responsive care is critical to brain development and positively affects children throughout their lives.

The care infants, toddlers, and preschool age children receive must vary based on the age of the child and their developmental stage. The elements of strength-based care build on each other as children move through their developmental milestones, supported by developmentally appropriate practices. Therefore, it is best to think of the elements of responsive caregiving in a more linear progression, helping one skill build upon another. The following table includes a sample of things infants and toddlers need in a responsive high-quality care setting.

TABLE 1.1. WHAT YOUNG CHILDREN NEED FROM THEIR CAREGIVERS

INFANTS AND TODDLERS *Caregivers use a calm, gentle, and nurturing manner to engage with young children.*	**PRESCHOOLERS** *Caregivers build on quality infant and toddler care to engage children through responsive care environment.*
They need us to • create soothing and calming environments that also provide novel and stimulating activities • quickly respond to their needs with gentle, soothing, and comforting facial expressions and tone of voice • respond in a positive and nurturing manner to their physical needs to be fed, rocked, soothed, and have their diapers changed • tune in to their signals to communicate with positive words, facial expressions, and actions • respond in ways that respect their individual needs • provide opportunities to freely play and explore • provide hands-on, multisensory experiences • provide opportunities for both indoor and outdoor exploration • create daily routines and provide a consistent, predictable learning environment • be sensitive to the individual differences in temperament and ability to adapt to change • be sensitive to sensory needs • provide love and nurturing care in the early learning environment	They need us to • help build their healthy brain connections through developmentally appropriate activities • provide novel activities so they can master new skills and develop new learning • integrate learning across all developmental domains: social, emotional, cognitive, language, and physical • create learning environments that provide structure, routines, and opportunities to explore and make choices • create quiet spaces where they can practice self-soothing and calming skills • design learning environments that allow for both large- and small-group instruction • encourage friendship-building skills through play and other social interactions • provide opportunities for early literacy development, including books and stories that teach social and emotional skills • scaffold opportunities to practice navigating social relationships individually and in groups • encourage their independence, initiative, and problem-solving skills

Because early brain development is so important to social and emotional development and wellbeing, it is discussed throughout this book. The early years provide caregivers with a window of opportunity to offer positive early experiences that will dramatically affect children's chances to build their sense of wellbeing. When we practice responsive caregiving, children's basic needs for loving, nurturing care are met and the child feels safe and secure. When caregivers respond in loving, nurturing ways, we are letting young children know that they are important to us and valuable to our classroom community, and that we understand what they are telling us and we respect their needs. As we approach early mental health and wellbeing, finding ways to support the whole child is important. Providing nurturing care in high-quality learning environments sets the landscape of social and emotional wellbeing.

High-Quality Early Learning Environments

As we explore the ways we support the emotional health and wellbeing of young children, we know that providing a high-quality early learning environment is essential. Although the world is rapidly changing, children continue to need food, shelter, comfort, cognitive stimulation, and emotional support. Feelings of trust, security, and love are still the cornerstone of future emotional wellbeing and mental health. During infancy, toddlerhood, and the preschool years, children learn through play, hands-on experiences, and the relationships with the adults who care for them and who support and scaffold their learning.

When examining early mental health and a child's state of wellbeing, we must consider the whole child and their social, emotional, cognitive, language, and physical development along the developmental continuum. As care providers, we know that social and emotional development can be integrated across all developmental domains. For example, as two or three children play together building with wood blocks, they are learning to share, play cooperatively, and form positive relationships with peers. When caregivers read books such as *I'm Happy-Sad Today: Making Sense of Mixed-Together Feelings* by Lory Britain or *That's What a Friend Is* by P.K. Hallinan to children, they bring social and emotional awareness through language and literacy (see appendix A for an extended list of books).

With a growing emphasis on high-quality early care settings, the National Association for the Education of Young Children (NAEYC) has set ten standards for early childhood programs (NAEYC 2005). These standards are recognized as best practices in quality care for young children. They are as follows:

- **Standard 1:** Relationships
- **Standard 2:** Curriculum
- **Standard 3:** Teaching
- **Standard 4:** Assessment of Child Progress
- **Standard 5:** Health
- **Standard 6:** Staff Competencies, Preparation, and Support
- **Standard 7:** Families
- **Standard 8:** Community Relationships
- **Standard 9:** Physical Environment
- **Standard 10:** Leadership and Management

These standards established by NAEYC are integrated throughout this book and in our understanding of early mental health and wellbeing in young children. High-quality care includes developmentally appropriate practices (DAP). Following DAP, a caregiver bases all instructional practices and decisions on these three things:

- theories of child development
- a child's individual strengths and needs, which are uncovered through authentic assessment
- a child's cultural background as defined by their community, family history, and family structure

In doing so, a caregiver nurtures a child's social, emotional, cognitive, language, and physical development. High-quality care adapts to the changing needs of children, families, and communities.

Prosocial values such as empathy, caring, sharing, compassion, and helping others are integrated into DAP and play-based activities. Prosocial values promote the development of social, emotional, physical, cognitive, and linguistic skills needed to navigate society as a whole. In high-quality programs, caregivers have an opportunity to plan activities that support prosocial values. These activities help to guild young children as they develop and strengthen relationships.

Guiding Young Children through Relationships

Many young children, including babies as young as six weeks of age, are spending the majority of their days in early childhood environments. Strong partnerships between parents and caregivers are critical to the healthy development and wellbeing of all children. Responsive caregivers partner with families, ensure secure attachments and relationships between adults and children, and assist children in acquiring skills across the learning domains, including social and emotional development. These skills foster a child's growing ability to identify, express, and regulate their emotions and to feel concern and empathy for others.

Caring and responsive caregivers help children develop and maintain a state of wellbeing—including health and happiness and building children's internal sense of meaning and purpose. Developing social and emotional skills in young children helps them build feelings of wellbeing. Many practitioners continue to view social and emotional development solely as curriculum, but it is more than that; it is based on authentic, respectful reciprocal relationships between a child and their peers, parents, and care providers. The relationships between a child and their caregivers provide opportunities for the child to develop who they are and find their place in the world. Responsive caregivers help children develop into people with a wide range of social and emotional competencies. Chapter 5 further discusses social and emotional development.

Concerns for children's mental health conditions and wellbeing often leave the adults caring for them wondering how best to support and assist the developing child. Learning to address the complex needs of children is part of a strength-based approach. Understanding both our own unmet needs as caregivers and the unmet needs of children is one facet of solution-based supports. Working as a primary caregiver requires a great deal both physically and emotionally. Early childhood environments are lively, noisy, and frequently very demanding places, and caregivers often feel overwhelmed and alone in managing the emotional needs of not just one child but an entire classroom of children. Across the nation, we are seeing more and more children demonstrating challenging and disruptive behaviors in the classroom environment. For example, caregivers are seeing children struggling to make and form friendships. Teachers report that they do not know how to respond to children's emotional outbursts. Even experienced teachers are voicing concerns and reporting stress in managing big emotions such as anger or rage in the classroom. Further, teachers are seeking guidance in supporting children who struggle with attention and self-control. Finally, we are hearing from the field that complex emotions are not limited to one child in a class but are occurring in rising numbers, thus increasing stress and safety concerns for both children and teachers in early childhood environments.

Increasingly complex emotional behaviors are surfacing in early learning settings, leading to three times the expulsion rate that is seen in K–12 schools (Gilliam 2005). NAEYC (2021) states, "Over a decade of research and data tell us that the policies and practices of suspension and expulsion in early childhood, which disproportionately affect children of color, are causing harm to children and families." Researchers further identified the decision factors for expulsion, including classroom disruption, fear of accountability, hopelessness, and teacher stress (Gilliam and Reyes 2018).

Rather than addressing concerning behaviors, many classrooms and programs simply label such students "problem children" and ask families to leave the program. But concerning behaviors are the outward actions or expressions of unmet needs. When we see children from a problem lens, we employ a deficit view of the child. We only identify the behavior, missing the child's unmet needs. Strength-based approaches look behind the curtain of the behavior to understand the underlying issues and needs.

If early care providers focus only on the outward behavior rather than the unmet need, children are apt to continue repeating the undesired action. Unmet needs can include the following:

- body needs—hunger, sleep, illness, or sensory overload
- emotional needs—consistent emotional supports, such as gentle touch, soothing, and comfort
- autonomy/control needs—control over the environment and ability to make choices
- developmental needs—developmentally appropriate and engaging experiences that allow for cognitive stimulation and exploration
- relational needs—trusting dyadic relationships with trusting adults and opportunities for peer interaction
- communication needs—being heard, recognized, respected, and valued

Children may also present or voice feelings of despair, hopelessness, helplessness, or inadequacy, and these too are expressions or signs of unmet needs.

As you work with children who show unmet needs through their behavior, continue to encourage and connect with them through small steps that build their confidence and relationships. To learn more about meeting the needs of the children in your care, we suggest you begin by examining the strength-based approach we call *Looking behind the Curtain* (see chapter 11 and QR codes for additional activities). In this approach, the *curtain* is the concerning behavior, and behind it is the child's unmet need or needs. Many providers only focus on the presenting behavior, or *curtain*.

It's important to remember that the children in our care are under the age of six and have limited life experiences and knowledge about social and emotional development. Because young children are still developing and understanding their needs and how to meet them successfully, they go about resolving them the best way they can. They are often overwhelmed by the intensity of their emotions, not knowing age-appropriate strategies for managing or regulating them. We also remember that young children more often communicate with their bodies than their words (Statman-Weil 2020). Unfortunately, in a classroom setting, children's attempts to meet their needs may be seen in these aggressive behaviors:

- fighting
- hitting
- biting
- destroying classroom or other children's property
- excessive crying
- clinging behavior
- throwing tantrums

Many times, if needs continue to be unmet, the behavior will escalate and become a safety issue for both children and caregivers. With the understanding that undesirable behaviors are unmet needs, guidance in the classroom then becomes how we change our reactions and engagement to help a child meet their needs.

Strength-based classrooms provide opportunities for children to learn age-appropriate ways to identify their needs and express themselves in safe, supportive environments. Our work, then, is to be aware of where a child might fall on the continuum of social and emotional to mental health so we can match the child's need with the supports that will best help them. When we separate needs from behaviors, we come to recognize that we do not seek to change undesirable behaviors but rather support the child in meeting their needs. As a responsive caregiver, remember that children need connection and a sense of belonging. The dyadic relationship becomes particularly important, since meeting an individual child's need happens in one-to-one engagement and not through group directions. You will see in both chapter 11 and the QR codes a variety of strength-based approaches and activities that will assist you as you design your classroom to help meet the needs and underlying issues of the children in your early learning environment.

We have learned that there is no one-size-fits-all approach to helping children regulate their emotions. What we do know is that it is imperative that we continue to educate our early childhood workforce about strength-based approaches and practices that can meet the changing needs of *all* children. In partnership with parents and families, caregivers have a critical role in supporting early interventions, promoting social and emotional development, and scaffolding safe, nurturing play-based environments.

Play

Play is a vital part of nurturing environments that guide young children. Play as a curriculum supports children's healthy brain development. For example, we know that play helps with executive function skills such as problem solving, identifying and regulating emotions, critical thinking, focus, and communication. Children benefit from all types of play. Research demonstrates direct correlations between play and children's social, emotional, cognitive, language, and physical growth, as well as moral development. Removing, limiting, or overstructuring children's play experiences can contribute to poor mental health outcomes. We believe that in high-quality early learning settings, play needs to be

- self-selected and self-directed by the child
- process based rather than goal based (as in sports)
- open-ended
- individually constructed
- encouraging imaginative exploration
- promoting curiosity with novel experiences
- building on prior knowledge and skills
- active rather than passive engagement
- embedded with opportunities for social engagement and building friendships

Play provides children with opportunities to build resiliency and develop creative problem-solving skills. Self-directed and open-ended play provides children with safe ways to express their feelings and concerns. By observing children's free play, caregivers can develop a broad and complex understanding of each individual child's developing strengths, competencies, and needs. Through play, children build confidence, developmental competencies, and relationship skills. Children's play and their sense of playfulness have a direct correlation to their ability to develop healthy social bonds with adults and peers. Children who lack sufficient exploratory play experiences may feel alone and isolated and lack the skills and confidence to initiate relationships. Therefore, they are often hesitant to try new experiences. Mental Health America identifies play as being as important as all other basic human needs, such as food, sleep, love, and acceptance. Play experiences stimulate the brain, offering young children opportunities to build on prior learning and develop and learn new skills. Play fosters collaboration, creativity, problem solving, and language skills, as well as focus and control.

In 1929 Mildred Parten identified six types of play, noting how a child's social skills are reflected in the way in which they engage in play (Parten 1932). Parten's identifications are still used today. It is important to note that Parten's age ranges can be somewhat fluid, and as children grow, they combine current and previous stages to create variation in their play experiences. The following are Parten's six types of play, linking each to its benefit to emotional wellness.

TABLE 1.2. PARTEN'S SIX TYPES OF PLAY

TYPE OF PLAY	DESCRIPTION	EMOTIONAL WELLNESS BENEFIT
Unoccupied Play *0 to 3 months*	In the first three months of life, children play through the exploration of their world. This play appears to be unorganized as young children explore materials around themselves (including their limbs).	Babies learn to explore their environment and make connections to objects through manipulation. Sensory input at this stage wires the first play connections in the brain, helping children to orient themselves in the world. It is the foundation of all play to follow.

Solitary (Independent) Play *3 months to 2.5 years*	Children younger than two years of age generally focus on a single activity or toy. Children work to develop mastery of the materials or activity through physical and cognitive action.	Children build confidence as they begin to develop and test theories about activities or objects. They learn to spend time with themselves as their cognitive processes begin to develop. Their confidence increases through autonomous actions.
Onlooker Play *2.5 to 3.5 years*	Onlooker play allows children to observe and then model play experiences. Children work out the physical movements of play, as well as the cognitive, social, and emotional structure of play.	In this stage, acts of listening and observing support a child's ability to understand what social interactions look like. As children observe others play, they begin to build a framework for their own wellbeing and compare their actions with others, and may even comment on what they see.
Parallel Play *3.5 to 4 years*	Parallel play builds on from onlooker play, as children now sit close to each other. They may begin to share resources but continue to focus on separate activities during play.	Learning to relate to others is fundamental in this type of play. Children build to make social connections.
Associate Play *4 to 4.5 years*	Children are engaged in play together and acknowledge one another, but it is not organized to a specific shared outcome. Rather, associate play demonstrates social engagement in parallel processes, such as children riding scooters next to each other or dancing to music.	Children are learning to navigate social experiences and begin to negotiate play materials. These early efforts of give and take begin to build on cooperative experiences.
Cooperative Play *4.5 years and up*	Children begin to work together in shared exchanges to collaborate toward a shared goal.	Social interactions are building as children learn to compromise to continue playing in a community. Different perspectives help young children to refine their ideas and actions.

Play is a universal human activity seen around the world in children of all ages. While play is universal, it is influenced by culture and looks different in different cultures. Cultural differences in play may include views based on these criteria:

- what is considered active versus aggressive
- what are acceptable risk levels
- what is considered gender appropriate
- what are considered acceptable noise levels
- how free play is valued
- who are acceptable play partners
- what types of play might occur and where play might take place

How might play vary between cultures? Let us look at one of the most common aspects of imaginative play: storytelling. Western European/US storytelling patterns strongly differ from those of other cultures. The most common Western European/US storytelling arc is *beginning, middle, end*. However, many other cultures do not follow this story arc. When observing children's play, identifying and evaluating storytelling patterns from our own cultural perspective is easy, as is identifying social and emotional development in children sharing our same cultural background. Research shows that when we observe play in other cultures, we often miss the complexity of the story lines and the social and emotional learning.

Caregivers are often not familiar with other cultures' patterns of storytelling, which leads to misinterpretation and underappreciation of children's development. Chapter 9 discusses expanding our interpretations of what we observe when working with children from cultures different than our own. As you examine the social and emotional landscape of wellbeing, pay careful attention to your own cultural norms when observing and documenting play experiences to assure that you are objectively interpreting what you are observing.

The Landscape of Social and Emotional Wellbeing

We know that a strong support system has many positive benefits for both children and their families. Our support system helps us develop coping and resiliency skills, scaffolds our learning, and gives us a positive, hopeful outlook on life. Support systems help us overcome many of life's challenges and obstacles while reducing feelings of anxiety and depression.

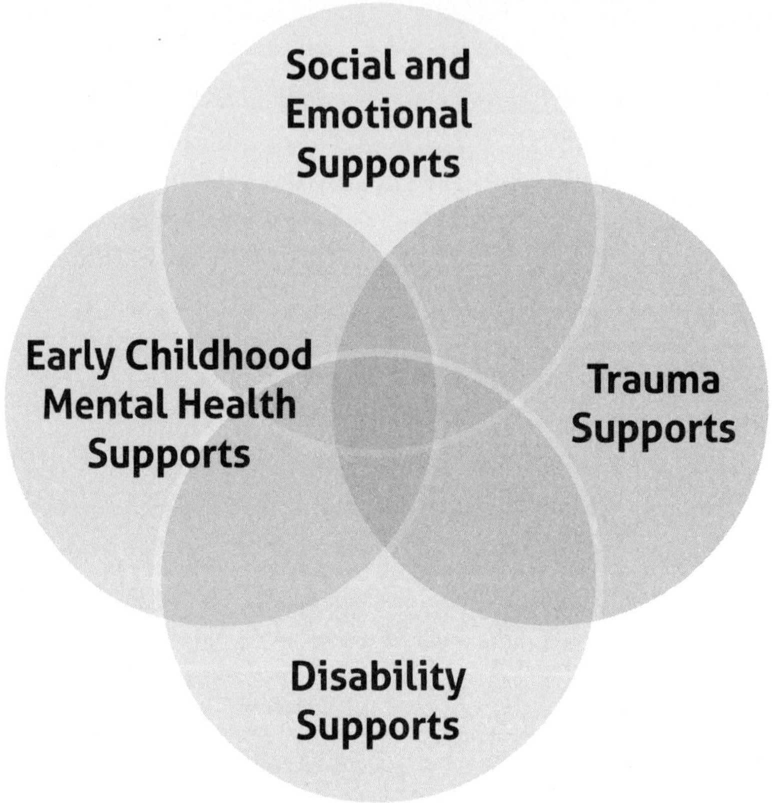

Figure 1.1. The Intersecting Needs for Support

There are four intersecting areas in which young children need support for their social and emotional development (see figure 1.1). As caregivers, we provide *social and emotional supports* to foster the development of typical skills needed for children to meet social and emotional developmental milestones.

Early learning settings need to provide multiple opportunities for children to learn and express their emotions in relationship with others. Trauma, disability, and early mental health supports are generally provided by specialists in their respective fields. Specialized *trauma supports* are needed for young children who have been or are being exposed to distressing or disturbing experiences over time that have rewired their brains. Trauma supports address the behaviors that emerge from trauma responses. *Disability supports* are provided for children who have a medical diagnosis, and for their families. A medical diagnosis can overlap with trauma and/or mental health. *Early childhood mental health supports* help children learn strategies for self-regulation, communication, and recognizing emotions in self and others. They are scaffolded experiences focused on promoting healthy social and emotional development for the parent-child dyad and can be extended to the early childhood setting or other caregivers. You will find opportunities to expand your knowledge of these four supports throughout the book.

TABLE 1.3. UNDERSTANDING THE INTERSECTING NEEDS FOR SUPPORT

TYPE OF SUPPORTS	WHAT ARE THE KEY IDEAS IN EACH SUPPORT SYSTEM?	WHAT TYPES OF SPECIALIZED SUPPORTS ARE AVAILABLE FOR CHILDREN AND FAMILIES?	WHAT ARE SOME EXAMPLES FROM YOUR PRACTICE?	WHAT DO YOU WANT TO LEARN MORE ABOUT?
Social and Emotional Supports				
Trauma Supports				
Disability Supports				
Early Childhood Mental Health Supports				

Overlap exists between support systems, and some children receive multiple services. Within each system, supports for children range from everyday best practices incorporated into every quality early childhood program to more complex, multisystem supports that include medical and mental health professionals. This book primarily focuses on early childhood mental health and its intersections with social and emotional and trauma supports.

THE FOUNDATIONS OF MENTAL HEALTH AND WELLNESS

Final Thoughts

The care and wellbeing of young children is an awesome responsibility for caregivers. Your role is understanding the complexity of the developing child and how strength-based approaches can set them on a positive trajectory toward mental health and wellbeing. As we have seen in this chapter, healthy play and social interaction are important for building relationships because reciprocal and respectful relationships between and among children, caregivers, and families help lay the foundation for long-term social and emotional wellness.

Taking Action

What Caregivers Can Do

- Identify strategies that promote relationship building between caregivers and children.
- List strength-based practices to support culturally inclusive classrooms.
- Describe the steps you can take to promote relationships and pro-social values in your classroom.

Reflection and Application

- What do respectful and reciprocal relationships look like with children and families?
- What are three ways you demonstrate that you are a responsive caregiver?
- How would you explain to families the importance of early brain development?

CHAPTER 2

Mental Health and Wellbeing

Mental health is a positive term that refers to the presence of mental or emotional wellness and the absence of mental illness.
—Carolina Amador, Inge Daeschel, and Joanne Sorte,
Nutrition, Health and Safety for Young Children: Promoting Wellness

Before beginning a closer examination of early mental health, we must first establish a solid understanding of the issues surrounding adolescent and adult mental health and the important role early education providers play in social and emotional development. Providing a solid foundation of social and emotional skills and a supportive living condition is important for all children. Youth ages ten to nineteen are experiencing many social, emotional, cognitive, language, and physical changes, further developing and maintaining social and emotional skills they acquired during early childhood. Skills such as making and maintaining friendships, showing empathy, regulating emotions, resolving conflict, and building resiliency are as important during the early years as they are in adolescence and in adulthood. These skills allow young children, as well as adolescents, to develop their sense of self and self-identity.

During the adolescent period of development, children are at risk for additional stress as they learn to form their own thoughts and opinions, question earlier beliefs, conform to peers and society, explore their sexual identity, and seek greater autonomy (Sorte, Daeschel, and Amador 2017). Increased use of technology and media can further pressure youth and decrease their ability to navigate realistic views of the world and society's expectations. Additionally, mental health outcomes can be influenced by exposure to violence, bullying, poverty, and abuse, making this age group especially vulnerable to mental health problems.

An adverse childhood experiences (ACEs) research study conducted between 1995 and 1997 by the Centers for Disease Control and Prevention (CDC) and 17,000 Kaiser Permanente patient volunteers found that both repeated or prolonged activation of a child's stress response without interventions by trusted, nurturing caregivers and living in an unsafe and unstable environment can lead to long-term changes in the structure and function of the brain and other biological changes (ACES Aware 2020). The study categorized adverse experiences in the domains of abuse, neglect, and childhood household dysfunction and demonstrated the cumulative effects on a child who has experienced toxic stress in any of the three domains. It found that ACEs were common among the study participants and that these experiences strongly related to various risk factors, causing serious health issues throughout their lifespans. Through its findings, the ACEs study indicates that effects of toxic stress are detectable as early as infancy. The ACEs findings leave us recognizing the importance of providing *all* children the opportunity to be cared for in a nurturing, responsive early learning environment that is safe, secure, and stable.

Mental Illness

Mental illness is a growing concern both in the United States and around the world. According to the World Health Organization (WHO), suicide is the third-largest cause of death for children ages fifteen to nineteen, and depression is one of the leading causes of illness and disability among adolescents worldwide (WHO 2019). According to the WHO, half of all mental health conditions begin by the time a child reaches age fourteen, and most cases go undetected or untreated. The National Alliance on Mental Illness (NAMI), the largest grassroots organization in the United States focused on improving the lives of Americans living with mental illness, provides advocacy, education, and support for people living with mental illness and their loved ones. NAMI also tracks mental illness statistics in the United States and in 2019 reported that one in five adults experiences a mental illness and one in twenty-five experiences a serious mental illness. These statistics help show how 20 percent of the population needs social and emotional supports. Wellbeing framed in this light then becomes of critical importance as we recognize that the children and families we serve may need supports. NAMI data showed that one in six children and youth between six and seventeen years old experience a mental health disorder each year. Both early supports and understanding young children's complex emotional needs are critical. With this alarming data, we are reminded of the importance of developing early social and emotional skills in young children and helping all children, youth, and adults feel safe, confident, and hopeful about the future. By examining mental health and mental illness, we can work together to provide early identification, support, education, and advocacy for individuals and families living with mental illness.

When mental health conditions go undetected or untreated, youth and young children are at greater risk for adult mental illness. Without early identification and proper treatment early in a child's life, children run the risk of impaired physical and mental health in adolescence and adulthood. With effective mental health services and supports, individuals develop close relationships with family and friends that help them lead happy, productive lives. Early childhood providers must support the social and emotional development of young children to provide them with the foundational skills necessary to navigate through adolescence and on to adulthood, skills that will last a lifetime.

Influences on Mental Health

Mental health and wellbeing are influenced by many factors, including prenatal care and gestation times, genetics, and environmental factors. Babies born before thirty-seven weeks of pregnancy are identified as preterm and are at increased risk for disabilities and neurological problems compared with children who are born at full term. Babies who are born with genetic anomalies, which may or may not have been identified before birth, may also need additional services and interventions. Other children are genetically predisposed to mental health issues or undiagnosed developmental delays that affect their overall health and wellbeing.

Additionally, prenatal care, including the mother's health, living conditions, and lifestyle choices, affects the developing fetus from conception throughout the child's life. A healthy lifestyle during and after pregnancy, good prenatal care and regular checkups with a medical professional, and stable living conditions positively influence the developing fetus, the newborn baby, and the growing child. When children are raised in a loving, nurturing, stable environment where the child's basic needs are met, they develop a sense of trust and security, learning that the world is a safe place. A lack of proper food, shelter, cognitive stimulation, or emotional care, as well as other disruptions in the developmental process, have the potential to negatively affect the child's social, emotional, cognitive, language, and physical development. We know that children who are exposed to traumatic events early in life are at risk for developing mental health issues. The severity of the living conditions, the frequency of exposure to traumatic events, and how the adults around them respond to and support children's responses to these events are critical. The presence of a consistent, secure adult in a child's life plays a critical role in how the child responds to traumatic events and how the event affects the child's developing state of mental health and wellbeing. Each adult who touches the life of a young child is responsible for treating them as individuals and honoring their uniqueness as people.

Mental Health versus Mental Illness

Mental health and mental illness are often grouped together or thought of as the same thing, but mental health and mental illness should be viewed as two separate dimensions. Mental health is an individual's psychological state of wellbeing, which includes satisfactory levels of social and emotional functioning, the ability to successfully adapt to and cope with normal life stressors, resiliency to events and changes in life, and age-appropriate behavior in both individual and social situations.

Mental illness is an illness and must be seen and treated as one. Mental illness can be defined as a wide range of conditions and disorders that affect an individual's behavior, mood, and thinking. A mental illness, also called a mental disorder or psychiatric disorder, is a combination of how a person feels, thinks, behaves, and perceives themselves and the world around them. For example, if a child has a diagnosed mental disorder or psychiatric disorder of depression, they exhibit a combination of symptoms, such as feelings of fatigue or loss of appetite, trouble focusing on tasks and following directions, and feelings of worthlessness, guilt, or self-blame. The diagnosis of a mental disorder is done by a mental health professional and meets specific criteria using a common diagnostic tool. The terms *mental illness* and *mental disorder* are used interchangeably throughout this book.

Mental illness includes a wide range of mental health disorders that cause significant impairment to an individual's daily living, interpersonal relationships, and personal functioning. Each mental health disorder consists of discrete symptoms or criteria that persist over time and do not improve on their own. Mental illness impacts an individual's mood, thinking, behavior, and ways of interacting with others. Mental disorders can greatly impair an infant's and young child's ability to learn and develop new skills. We examine mental health disorders commonly recognized in early childhood in chapter 7.

Early diagnosis and treatment of mental illness are essential to allowing young children to form healthy social and emotional skills. Some young children are diagnosed before age five, while others are diagnosed later in elementary school or high school as their levels of daily functioning, interpersonal relationships, and behaviors change. In young children, symptoms of mental disorders may include difficulties in how they learn, speak, act, play with others, focus, attend to adults and activities, and regulate their emotions. Sometimes behaviors in young children are isolated and need not cause concern. We must consider not only the symptoms but also the age of the child and the length of time symptoms have been present.

To better understand mental disorders in young children, we must become familiar with the types of diagnostic tools used by mental health professionals. The *American Psychiatric Association: Diagnostic and Statistical Manual of Mental Disorders*, 5th edition (DSM-5) is a common tool in the United States used by clinicians, medical professionals, and researchers to understand and diagnose mental disorders. The DSM-5 uses a lifespan approach to mental health, beginning with infancy. It does not isolate childhood conditions but recognizes that conditions may manifest at different stages of life and be influenced developmentally along a continuum. Similar to the DSM-5, the *International Classification of Diseases*, 10th edition (ICD-10), maintained by the World Health Organization, is used internationally as a diagnostic tool for health management, epidemiology, and mental health purposes.

For the purposes of this book, we will discuss mental disorders using the *Diagnostic Classification of Mental Health and Developmental Disorders of Infancy and Early Childhood DC:0–5* (Zero to Three 2016). Based on emerging data and research in 2016, Zero to Three updated and revised the previous *Diagnostic Classification of Mental Health and Developmental*

Disorders of Infancy and Early Childhood DC:0–3R with DC:0–5. It was not designed to compete with or replace the DSM-5 or the ICD-10, but to further identify syndromes that are unique to children from birth through age five. DC:0–5 differs from the other two diagnostic manuals by placing careful consideration on early child development, developmental disorders, the importance of early caregiving relationships, and the role of attachment in early mental disorders. DC:0–5 is an age-specific tool that classifies early mental health and developmental disorders within the context of families, cultures, and communities.

Universally recognized diagnostic guides such as the DSM-5, ICD-10, and DC:0–5 are useful because they give clinicians, medical professionals, and researchers standard language and descriptive classifications of disorders, allowing them to clearly communicate presenting issues and design appropriate treatment plans. A common nosology, or list of classified disorders, helps professionals connect individuals and their families to a broad range of support services.

Mental Health Considerations

The diagnosing of mental health disorders is a complex process. The process allows professionals working with the child and family to consider the child's presenting symptoms as they diagnose and create an effective diagnostic treatment plan. We know that mental health and wellbeing are strongly influenced by a variety of factors, including the relationship between the child and their primary caregiver, a reciprocal relationship in which optimally both parent(s) and child play an active role. The caregiving environment and caregiver's contribution are assessed in many ways, including the following:

- the child's basic needs for food, clothing, and shelter are being met
- there is a positive emotional investment on the part of the caregiver(s)
- the child's physical health is maintained
- the child is provided comfort and has consistent feelings of safety and security
- the child receives age-appropriate socialization and cognitive stimulation
- the child receives age-appropriate behavioral guidance
- there are routines and structure in the home

- the child's temperament and learning style is taken into consideration
- the child's strengths and needs are recognized by caregiver(s)

Additionally, the clinician will assess whether there are psychosocial or environmental stressors contributing to the child's presenting symptoms, such as the death of a parent, a change in living situations, domestic violence in the home, mental illness of a parent or caregiver, the presence of emotional or physical abuse, substance abuse in the home, or local or community violence.

Clinicians also consider developmental milestones when they are assessing a child for mental disorders. Typically recognized milestones are broken into age ranges, beginning with birth to three months and progressing through age five. How the child reaches or meets developmental milestones helps a clinician determine next steps, including making a diagnosis and designing a treatment plan. For you the caregiver, assessing children's growth along a developmental continuum helps you share your concerns with parents and mental health professionals. How the child adapts and varies their behavior in differing environments provides valuable information for the clinician. Using a research-based developmental screening tool is considered a best practice in the field of early education. When consistent patterns of behavior begin to emerge, clinicians can better assess the strengths and difficulties the child presents.

Once an infant or young child is diagnosed with a disorder, a team of professionals, which may include nurses, physical and occupational therapists, or speech pathologists, among others, work together to provide comprehensive services for the child and their family. Each state has its own licensing requirements that identify which professionals may diagnose and treat individuals. Page 32 has a list of the mostly commonly recognized professionals who diagnose and form treatment and prevention plans.

TABLE 2.1. PROFESSIONAL MENTAL HEALTH PRACTITIONERS AND SPECIALISTS

TITLE	EDUCATION	EXPERIENCE
Early Interventionist	Master's degree	Provides specialized interventions and diagnosis for children ages 0–5 years; may be a physical therapist, occupational therapist, or speech therapist
Licensed Mental Health Counselors (LMHC)	Master's degree	Provides mental, behavioral, and emotional health counseling to individuals, families, and groups
Licensed Marriage and Family Therapists (LMFT)	Master's degree	Provides psychotherapy and family system work with individuals and families experiencing mental health and emotional problems; clinical experience in marriage and family therapy
Licensed Master Social Worker (LMSW)	Master's degree	Works with individuals and families to improve social and health outcomes and obtain appropriate services to resolve social and health problems
Licensed Clinical Social Worker (LCSW)	Master's degree	Licensed to provide psychotherapy to help individuals with a variety of mental health and daily living conditions, with clinical experience in marriage and family therapy
Psychologist (PhD or PsyD)	Doctoral degree in psychology	Licensed in clinical psychology with specialized skills in mental health working with children, adolescents, adults, couples, and families
Psychiatrist (MD or DO)	Medical degree	A medical physician who specializes in mental health and can prescribe and monitor medications

Final Thoughts

As interpersonal relationships are so central to a child's development and wellbeing, your role in helping children feel loved and connected to others is critically important. Informing parents when you become concerned about the child's developmental trajectory is helpful in the early detection of disorders. We know that early detection and interventions for mental disorders and developmental delays greatly influence the developing brain and have a positive impact on the child's overall developmental trajectory. In this chapter, we provided background knowledge in the distinctions between mental health and mental illness. Understanding the complexity of mental wellbeing is critical to your work in identifying typical milestones across all developmental domains.

Taking Action

What Caregivers Can Do

- Become familiar with the difference between mental health and mental illness.
- Understand what influences mental health and wellbeing.
- Understand children's social and emotional needs in early care environments.
- Understand the roles and types of mental health professionals.

Reflection and Application

- What do I need to know about mental health and wellness to support young children in my care?
- What steps can I take to identify mental health professionals in my community?
- What information can I learn about ACEs to be able to recognize risk factors in children and families?

CHAPTER 3

Caregiver Wellbeing

We care for ourselves to be in care of others.
—Mandy Davis, Trauma Informed Oregon

The emotional lives of children and caregivers come together in classrooms in meaningful and authentic ways. We choose careers in early childhood because we are drawn to working with young children and desire to make a positive, lasting impact on their lives. Supporting young children in their development is deeply personal. Your commitment and dedication to helping children engage in their first interactions with individuals outside of their immediate families is commendable.

Every day, the early learning environment is filled with both the children's and our own emotions. Planning for the emotional climate in the classroom involves more than curriculum; it involves our own emotional preparation. Emotional preparation (discussed later in this chapter) helps us ready our brains and bodies to work. Once emotionally prepared to work, we are able to make ourselves emotionally available to the children. While much of our day is spent supporting children's overall development, including social and emotional development, very little attention is given to our emotional needs as caregivers. Why is this important? New research shows that our emotional health as primary caregivers is linked to the emotional health of children. This is because children form attachments with their primary caregivers, and early attachment greatly influences future mental health and wellbeing not just now, but for a lifetime. This chapter focuses on caregiver wellbeing and how we prepare to work with young children in emotionally healthy ways.

Understanding Caregiver Wellbeing

As early childhood caregivers, we spend a significant amount of time developing the skills needed to teach and provide optimal care for the children in our early learning environments. We learn to work with children in a variety of ways, striving to meet the needs of each individual. Our goal is to help them both reach their full social, emotional, and academic potential, and feel safe, healthy, and nurtured. Each day is different and requires constant change, with its own physical, mental, and emotional pressures.

The term *emotional labor* is used when a job or profession requires emotional regulation while working with others. It includes displaying a set of emotions appropriate for the situation and not displaying emotions when they are inappropriate. We are required to manage our feelings, yet also express them daily in our work with young children. In fact, without the expression of feelings, we are unable to make the relational connections that are the foundation of children's learning and our own emotional wellbeing. When a child is tearful and looks to you for comfort, acknowledge their feelings and their need for security and comfort. Verbally assure them while standing or sitting close to them. Your actions need to convey closeness and reassurance to the child. Their attachment to you and your authentic relationship with them offers a sense of security and trust. As caregivers, helping a child name and manage their feelings while keeping our own emotions in check is important, even when we are tired or frustrated.

Working in our field places many demands on our emotions; therefore, we need to carefully honor our own time and energy along with the needs of the children and their families. Think of yourself as a pitcher of milk—you are constantly pouring milk from the pitcher, filling drinking glasses by attending to the emotions of others and yourself. At some point, the pitcher becomes empty. Thinking about how you "fill your pitcher" is important. Do you work out at the gym, read a good book, or meet a friend for coffee?

All the nurturing things you do for yourself help you replenish your "pitcher" and become more emotionally resilient.

Maintaining a balance between our time and energy increases our emotional resiliency (see Developing a Self-Care Plan on page 41). Our emotional resiliency is strengthened not only when we take time for ourselves outside of work but also when we have the skills to do our work and the time to engage in planning and reflective practices. Dr. Dan Siegel coined the term *window of tolerance* to refer to our ability to tolerate the ups and downs of not only our own emotions but the emotions of others (Attachment and Trauma Treatment Center 2020). Developing emotional resiliency helps us to understand our own window of tolerance and thus combats burnout. Burnout occurs when we must expend emotional energy in our work but have no way to replace it.

Developing emotional resiliency requires us to pay attention to our own state of wellbeing. Wellbeing for adults in early childhood education is much more than just physical health; it also includes social, emotional, and cognitive health. Wellbeing in early care providers also includes a positive sense of self and a clear purpose to make a difference in the lives of young children. In early childhood care environments, this sense of self and purpose come from thinking deeply about our practice. While we work in early childhood because we love children, we must go beyond this surface analysis to deeply understand why this work is important to us.

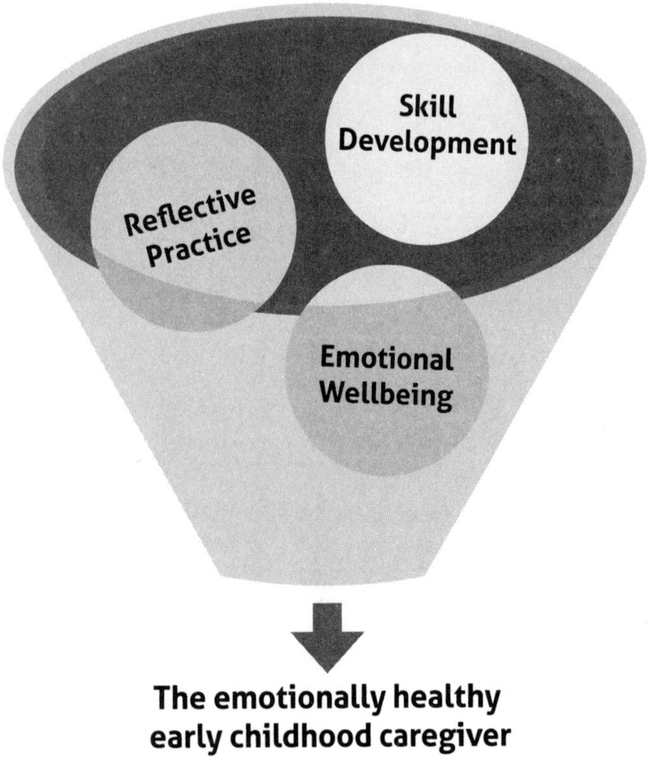

Practices for Emotional Health

In early childhood education, caregiver wellbeing is based on three elements: skill development, reflective practice, and emotional wellbeing (see figure 3.1). Each element

Figure 3.1. The Three Elements of Caregiver Wellbeing

The emotionally healthy early childhood caregiver

supports a different function of the caregiver's role and the high-quality care they provide in their classroom.

Skill Building

Skill development includes all the basic skills necessary to effectively provide high-quality care while successfully working with young children. These skills encompass an understanding of child development and knowledge of developmental competencies, along with skills in navigating the early childhood environment. They include the following:

- knowledge of different theories of child growth and development
- ability to prepare developmentally appropriate learning environments and play-based curriculum
- knowledge of culture and families
- ability to address the health, safety, and nutritional needs of young children
- skills to observe, assess, and reflect on children's lives in the classroom and plan strategic interventions for optimal growth and development
- ability to manage the classroom or program to meet the legal and business practices of early childhood programs
- skills to provide supports for young children with disabilities to fully integrate them into classrooms and programs
- ability to support young children's emotional health and build classroom community through the understanding of children's social and emotional experiences and expressions
- desire to improve skills and engage in professional growth

The skills in the areas listed are considered necessary—they constitute best practice in the field of early childhood education and are foundational to what we know and do when working with children birth through age five. No matter if you have worked in the field for many years or are just starting out, basic knowledge and skills in these areas are essential to being a resilient practitioner. Without basic skill development, we face unnecessary struggles that erode our sense of wellbeing and impair our feelings of confidence, lowering our ability to respond effectively to the children in our care. As we continue to mature in our practice, our foundational skills deepen through a combination of professional development, experience, and personal reflection.

Reflective Practice

Reflective practice is demonstrated through personal, focused reflection on our emotional health and wellbeing and on our adult-child relationships and caregiving practice. Internal reflective practice includes how we take care of our social, emotional, cognitive, and physical needs. When we focus on our emotional health, we increase our self-awareness. In particular, learning from the moments when we feel strong emotions such as frustration, discouragement, joy, and accomplishment helps us self-regulate and understand our emotional triggers. Reflecting on what we feel and why increases our resiliency. When we are aware of what triggers our emotions, we identify our emotional states faster. The sooner we are aware of what we are feeling, the sooner we can begin to regulate our emotions. Our ability to pause and reset our emotional climate greatly decreases the stress we feel during the day.

Professional reflective practice deals with the emotions that arise from the complexity of our work with young children. As caregivers we need to ask ourselves, *Why is it important to understand the difference between our personal and professional emotions?* The decisions we make need to be based on professional standards. Often issues regarding young children's behaviors and our emotional responses to these behaviors bump up against our personal values rather than our professional ones. Individual personal values are as unique as you are. When our personal values are challenged by another human being's actions, we respond from those personal values rather than our professional ones. Therefore, professional values, as outlined in NAEYC's Code of Ethical Conduct, are so important to making decisions about caregiving. They reflect a universal expectation that professional decisions are based on a justifiable professional course of action.

Professional reflective practice helps us to think through our personal and professional values and identify and examine the emotions that arise from our work as caregivers. For example, think about a time in the classroom that felt particularly frustrating or joyful. What went well? What did not go well? What could you do again or do differently? Asking these questions allows us to understand what was happening when we felt particular emotions. This understanding helps us become more aware of our feelings and how to modify or continue our interactions and improve our practice.

Skipping the self-reflection part of our professional practice can be tempting, since at the end of a long day, taking this extra time can be difficult. But much like cleaning the classroom, we must also check in with ourselves and process the emotions that emerged. Both actions prepare us to work with children and evaluate what we might change so the next day will go well. The following are stages of reflective practice that will assist you in adding self-reflection to your work with young children and increasing your sense of wellbeing.

TABLE 3.1. STAGES OF REFLECTIVE PRACTICE

	UNDERSTANDING	**REFLECTION**	**CRITICAL REFLECTION**
Personal Reflections *Journals, video blogs, notes, images, etc.*	Learning to identify what we see and feel when we teach; coming to understand the emotions that we feel throughout the day	Separating what we think and feel, interpreting what we see	Reflecting deeply on what is seen; asking open-ended questions, feeling comfort with disequilibrium and uncertainty in the outcome of questions
Professional Reflections *Journals, daily pages, observational notes, running records, etc.*	Reflecting on what we see, hear, and experience	Using a protocol to extend thinking and ask open-ended questions that unpack ideas	Challenging assumptions, considering multiple perspectives, asking complex questions, and allowing for not knowing answers

Reflection follows a developmental process. We develop our reflective capability like we develop muscles in our body. It takes time to build our practice. Our reflective capacity grows over time when we strive to make sense of our own and others' emotions, those of children and colleagues alike. Reflective practice helps us make sense of our own behaviors and those of others by increasing our understanding of the needs behind the behaviors. Concerning behavior is the face of unmet needs. Reflective practice allows us to understand what is behind our own feelings. Until we understand our own motivations, understanding the feelings behind young children's actions remains difficult.

Emotional Wellbeing

Emotional health encompasses the practices we use to recognize and understand our emotional states and regulate our emotions. For early childhood educators, emotional skills are the skills and activities that help minimize the sense of isolation that often occurs in the work of early childhood education. Further, these skills allow us to navigate boundaries, establish compassionate and self-compassionate practices, and engage in self-care that leads to healthy relationships. Caregivers develop their emotional skills through a deep understanding of their own emotional health and wellbeing. Social and emotional skills in caregivers include the knowledge, attitudes, and ability in early childhood settings to:

- accurately identify what we are feeing
- understand our emotional states during the course of our day
- regulate our emotions
- establish and maintain positive relationships with children and other adults in the classroom
- identify our personal versus professional values and make responsible decisions
- control our personal and professional emotions in our work
- set and achieve developmentally appropriate goals for young children
- set boundaries and practice healthy self-care

Emerging research identifies self-sacrifice as one of the traits of caregiving professionals that can diminish professional boundaries. Lacking clarity between "who I am and what I do" (Osgood 2012) leads to blurred personal and professional boundaries. This entanglement of the personal and professional selves reinforces personal attributes of altruism that foster a professional belief in the importance of self-sacrifice as a requirement of the work (Osgood 2012). A lack of strong professional boundaries decreases our emotional resiliency and ability to bounce back from the emotional labor of teaching.

Professional boundaries are fundamental to emotional wellness. Engaging in emotionally healthy activities supports our emotional regulation. Activities can range from hobbies to athletics, from meeting with friends to going to movies—the things we enjoy doing on our own or with others. These activities provide opportunities for our bodies and minds to rest and relax, bringing our lives into a state of balance and restoring our mindset so we can optimally care for and nurture the children in our learning environments.

Without time for all three—skills development, reflective practice, and activities that support emotional wellbeing—we risk burnout in our jobs (Osgood 2012). The early childhood field has many challenges that affect our emotional wellbeing, including long hours, low pay, lack of professional supports, and highly structured, outcomes-driven educational models in the early years. All of these elements can wear us down and decrease our resiliency in working with children. The less resilient we are, the harder it is to be emotionally present in the classroom. We can increase our resiliency by developing self-care plans.

Developing a Self-Care Plan

Self-care plans support our wellbeing. Rather than a list you need to complete, a self-care plan is a reflection of what you value and need in your daily, weekly, monthly, and yearly life to be emotionally healthy. Self-care plans allow us to reflect on what we value and ensure that self-care is part of our everyday lives.

Step 1: Reflect on activities you value and that give you moments of joy throughout the day, such as a hug from a loved one or a simple treat. ***What brings you joy in your daily life?***

Step 2: Think about activities that bring joy or happiness but may not happen every day, such as seeing a favorite friend, taking a vacation, or learning something new. ***What brings you joy over time?***

Step 3: Focus on the different domains of life: social, emotional, cognitive, physical, psychological, and professional. As you think about these domains, make a list, create a web, or otherwise write down what you are doing to take care of yourself in each area.

Physical: Taking care of your body, from exercising to healthy eating to sleeping, including scheduling medical and dental visits and attending to personal grooming.

Cognitive: Keeping your mind active outside of work, including reading, hobbies, art, gardening, playing music, and any other activities that engage your imagination. This can also include attending concerts, visiting museums or other places of interest, and engaging in new experiences.

Social: Investing in healthy relationships by spending time with and giving attention to those who are important to you, including supporting and nurturing these relationships by remembering special dates and connecting over important events.

Emotional: Knowing and recognizing your inner life. Connecting your feelings to your experiences. Expressing thoughts and emotions in ways that are healthy for yourself and others. Connecting with those who are emotionally healthy for you. Thinking about your self-talk by celebrating your achievements and practicing self-compassion with your mistakes.

Psychological: Taking care of your own emotional health, including self-care and practicing reflection or mindfulness, which can include journaling, meditation, developing new skills, or spending time with yourself without distractions.

Professional: Balancing your professional and personal lives by not sacrificing one for the other. Setting boundaries with tasks and people. Also includes investing in yourself and your skill set, and practicing time management and future planning.

Step 4: Review your list. Reflect on the areas where you are doing well and on those you value that might be missing from your daily, weekly, or monthly life.

Step 5: Remembering that a self-care plan is not a to-do list, think about how and where you might add things that will positively contribute to your quality of life. Reflect on how you might begin adding more self-care to your life. Start small and be sure to revisit your thinking to continue taking care of yourself.

Emotional Regulation in the Classroom

New research points to the biological connection between our emotional state and those of the children we teach (Lipscomb et. al. 2021). Studies of stress responses, measured by the stress hormone cortisol, show that if early childhood caregivers experience stress, then the children in their care can experience elevated stress. Stressful early learning environments decrease both children's and adults' sense of wellbeing. The quality of the program also affects stress levels in children and their caregivers. Additional biomarkers, or measurements of physical states of being, such as cortisol levels, breathing, and even heartbeats, can be correlated with attunement between children and caregivers, as these can sync together when there is a strong connection between caregiver and child.

This attunement to each other can be seen when we engage in serve-and-return behaviors or make connections during caregiving activities that strengthen the dyadic relationship. For example, a baby smiles and the caregiver responds by smiling back. This continues back and forth, and the extended interaction creates the serve-and-return response. Attunement supports adults and children in responding to each other's emotional rhythms. Caregivers who are attuned to the individual needs of each child read each child's emotional cues and supportively respond to them. The child responds back to the adult, who responds back to the child, and so on. We see this in practice when we are telling a story and are completely focused on the experience, then look up and see that all the children have also stilled and are focused.

Classroom environments that are based on mutual respect look very different from dysregulated classrooms. We have all experienced walking into a classroom where its noise and energy instinctually felt chaotic. In these dysregulated spaces, there is rarely the quiet hum of children engaged in self-directed work. Rather, children are not playing cooperatively, they have difficulty solving problems on their own, or they may be wandering around the classroom not knowing where to begin playing.

There are many reasons for dysregulated classrooms, such as routines being either lacking or inflexible; children being expected to follow excessive or unrealistic rules; or adults being burned out, over ratio, or unsupported. In dysregulated classrooms, the voices, actions, or behaviors of one child or a few children significantly affect the class as a whole. Classroom management moves from the dyadic interaction between an individual child to an environment where the caregiver just tries to maintain order throughout the day. Attempting to influence an individual child's voice, actions, or behaviors through whole-group controls, such as reminding, coaxing, doing things for the child that they can do themselves, or removing the child from the area, rarely succeeds. Thus, the children, caregivers, or both feel stressed and emotionally off balance. Caregivers in these spaces feel like they are always in crisis management. Once a classroom is dysregulated, both the children and the adults experience elevated levels of cortisol and stress, which also affect the social and emotional health of the classroom and often lead to increases in children's atypical social behaviors. This in turn leads to caregivers' decreased ability to lead from a place of emotional health and creates a spiral effect of crisis that increases with each further incident.

Emotionally healthy caregivers are more equipped to deal with the everyday challenges of teaching in early childhood classrooms. Their classrooms focus on respectful reciprocal relationships, valuing the contributions of every member of the classroom community. Healthy classroom communities also correlate to biomarkers that demonstrate lowered levels of stress and, in turn, increased readiness to learn. We like to say that if a child's brain is in a regulated, calm, and relaxed state, then the brain is ready to learn.

Caregivers' Emotional Worlds

Responsive caregivers are emotionally available to meet the daily challenges of early childhood learning environments. The child-caregiver dyad is the foundation of respectful reciprocal relationships, and dyadic relationships do not work unless caregivers are in an emotional state of wellbeing. To be emotionally ready and available for the work, we need to understand how our personal and professional experiences affect our emotions and ability to self-regulate each day.

Emotion Preparedness

Your emotional state and your internal emotional climate prior to entering the classroom determine how present and available you are to the children in your setting. Your emotional readiness to teach is affected by a variety of factors, including the relationships and events around you both at home and at work. For example, if you did not sleep well the night before work, you might be tired and more irritable, or if you had a disagreement with someone at home, you might be distracted at work. Making every effort to leave outside distractions at the classroom door can greatly improve your emotional state as a care provider. We all understand that this can be difficult to do. Here we offer some suggestions that can enhance your emotional preparedness and increase your resiliency:

- Practice self-care (taking care of self).
- Embrace self-compassion (forgive yourself for mistakes).
- Take actions that reinforce work/life balance.
- Engage in activities to increase emotional preparedness.
- Look for experiences that reinforce positive emotions.
- Work to eliminate experiences that lead to negative emotions and feelings.
- Reflect on everyday practices that help you center yourself.

Emotional Availability

Our work requires our emotional availability so we can connect with children in a loving and caring manner. Emotional availability includes skills and actions such as active listening, reciprocal exchanges, coming in close proximity to children to talk to them, being at their eye level, and expressing their emotions to them through words. We are emotionally available to children when we respond to children's joy by expressing joy ourselves in their learning and discoveries. Expressing joy to each other is a foundation of building trust. Recognizing joy in one another is one of the most authentic shared emotions between children and caregivers.

Emotional Temperature

We read our emotional temperature by recognizing our own range of emotions and understanding what triggers them and checking in with how we are emotionally feeling and how we are responding to the demands of children throughout the day. Your emotional availability also determines your emotional temperature as you help children regulate their range of emotions.

Taking your emotional temperature throughout the day will help you navigate the ups and downs of your program's emotional climate. Ask yourself questions such as, *Is my emotional pitcher empty or full?* or *Are the children's behaviors making me mad or angry, or am I feeling calm, relaxed, and ready to help?* Take ten minutes or so before you start your day to sit quietly without distractions and center yourself. In this quiet time, allow feelings to come up. Acknowledge their presence before you let them go. This simple reflective act will allow you to be more present when you enter your classroom.

Supporting Caregiver Emotional Health

Many times we feel emotionally drained by our work as caregivers. Knowing our emotional temperature allows us to recognize these feelings. Here are some warning signs that you are beginning to feel fatigued or burned out:

- recurring feelings of frustration or resentment toward children, parents, or coworkers
- irritability and impatience with the children
- feelings of vulnerability and sadness, such as tearfulness
- inability to control temper or outbursts of anger

- apathy toward actively engaging with the children or adults
- singling out one child as the focus of your frustration and outbursts
- not wanting to go to work or poor work attendance
- failing to plan for your daily instruction
- inflexibility in interactions with others, including an inability to change routines, activities, or environments
- meeting your emotional needs through unhealthy choices (anything to excess)

The field of early childhood education requires a lot from us, both physically and emotionally. At some point in our work lives, most early childhood caregivers experience what we call compassion fatigue. Similar to burnout, compassion fatigue is the state when our sense of compassion for others decreases over time. When we experience compassion fatigue, we focus on negative emotions like feeling helpless, depressed, and less hopeful. We may experience physical symptoms such as depression, stress, or anxiety. Our personal and professional lives are affected as we experience increased self-doubt, lack of focus, or decreased productivity (Day and Anderson 2011). At points of vulnerability or low resiliency, we are more sensitive to the actions of others, including parents and coworkers. These are periods where your pitcher is low or even empty altogether. If compassion fatigue is left unresolved, caregivers can feel emotionally hijacked, as though someone else is dictating their emotions. We know that we cannot control the actions of others, so we therefore need to take steps to support and build up our resiliency. We can do this through reflective practices and healthy relationships with friends, family, and coworkers who are supportive of our emotional wellbeing.

We can begin to observe and address feelings of burnout and compassion fatigue through self-awareness, daily temperature reading, and reflective practices. Other ways to address these feelings are keeping a balance between work and home, maintaining a strong network of friends outside of work that encourage and support you, setting strong boundaries with friends and family, and feeling a healthy sense that the work you do with children will have a lasting impact on their lives.

Final Thoughts

We strengthen our resiliency by keeping our emotional pitchers filled. We identify what skills we need, reflect on our practices, and take time to address our own emotional wellbeing. Emotionally healthy caregivers are more resilient and able to bounce back when faced with challenging situations. In addition to understanding our daily emotional temperature, acknowledging and addressing our emotional preparedness and availability to do the work is also important. Being sensitive to our emotions and what triggers them is another important component to a healthy classroom environment founded on respectful reciprocal relationships.

Taking Action

What Caregivers Can Do

- Keep a journal or log of your emotions during the day. Which parts of the day bring up positive or negative emotions?
- Use reflective practices throughout the day to learn to understand your emotional state of wellbeing and what behaviors trigger you.
- Create and post a self-care plan in your classroom where you can regularly refer to it.

Reflection and Application

- What fills your pitcher? How do you evaluate your work-life balance to keep your pitcher filled?
- How do you prepare yourself for the day? What routines do you create or actions do you take to be emotionally available for children?
- What additional skills do you need to support your emotional resiliency in your work?

CHAPTER 4

The Six Pillars of Strength-Based Caregiving

Whoever influences the child's life ought to try to give him a positive view of himself and of his world. The child's future happiness and his ability to cope with life and relate to others will depend on it.
—Bruno Bettelheim

Respectful, responsive caregiving based in children's and families' strengths is founded upon the dyadic relationship, the individualized relationship between one child and one caregiver. This chapter gives an overview of the Six Pillars of strength-based caregiving and how they work together to promote the mental health and wellbeing of children ages birth through five. Similar to pillars that create a building's solid structure, the Six Pillars provide the support for child wellbeing through strength-based caregiving and respectful reciprocal relationships that meet young children's needs. This practice can be simply defined as a child receiving everything they need to thrive.

The Research behind the Six Pillars Framework

The Six Pillars of strength-based caregiving emerge from the dyadic relationship between child and caregiver. The concept of dyadic relationships gained traction in the infant mental health field when researchers began studying attachment between parent (primarily the mother) and child. Since the 1980s, the quality of attachment and the dyadic relationship between mother and child have been measured through socioemotional milestones developed by the researchers Greenspan and Wieder (as cited in Lillas and Turnbull 2009):

- Milestone 1—Attention and regulation (birth–3 months)
- Milestone 2—Mutual engagement and attachment (3–6 months)
- Milestone 3—Purposeful, two-way communication (4–10 months)
- Milestone 4—Complex gestures and problem solving (10–18 months)
- Milestone 5—Use of symbols to express thoughts and feelings (18–30 months)
- Milestone 6—Bridges between symbols and emotional themes (30–48 months)

Lillas and Turnbull (2009) explain how dyadic relational interactions became a tool of measurement for the *DC 0–3: Diagnostic Classification of Mental Health and Developmental Disorders of Infancy and Early Childhood,* revised (1994, 2005). When the DC 0–3 was first released, it was the standard for age-specific assessment of young children by professional mental health practitioners and specialists (see table 2.1). In 2016 the classification tool was expanded to include diagnostic classifications for all young children zero to five years. The DC:0–5 classifies mental health and development disorders in young children up to the age of five years within the context of their families, cultures, and communities. Caregivers need a general knowledge of the mental health disorders more commonly seen in our early care settings in order to assist mental health practitioners in promoting children's mental health and wellbeing (discussed in chapter 7).

We developed the Six Pillars based on new research that has emerged over the past decade. What has become evident is that young children attach to their caregivers in addition to their parents, particularly when they attend full-day programs. Since young children are developing feelings of attachment to both their parent and the early childhood caregiver, each attachment significantly affects their healthy social and emotional development. No longer is the early childhood caregiver seen as a secondary support. They serve a primary role in the fundamental development of social and emotional health outside the home. We discuss attachment in greater detail in chapter 6.

Our new knowledge changes the relationship and role between young children and their early care providers. Caregivers now need the skills to develop and sustain a healthy dyadic relationship with each individual child, in addition to relationships in the larger classroom community. While caregivers support all children in their classroom, respectful reciprocal relationships are developed individually by spending quality time with each child to develop unique relationships and healthy attachments that meet their particular needs. Dyadic relationships play a significant role in how a young child's brain is wired and grows across all domains—socially, emotionally, cognitively, linguistically, and physically.

The Six Pillars of Strength-Based Caregiving

The Six Pillars provide the foundation for child wellbeing through the strength-based approaches to the dyadic relationship between the individual child and the individual caregiver. To develop a strength-based approach, caregivers need foundational skills to address the complex and sometimes challenging work of supporting young children's development. Here are some of these skills:

- recognizing young children's social and emotional development and health
- applying knowledge to support attachment through the dyadic relationship
- interpreting children's behaviors correctly and identifying supports along the mental health continuum
- identifying the unmet needs that lead to children's concerning behaviors and identifying risks and resiliency in each child
- constructing relationships with families that honor each family's unique strengths and culture
- analyzing your own role and that of others to provide referrals and supports for families

Together these skills are the foundation of a practice using a strength-based approach. The Six Pillars of strength-based caregiving will help you build your skills by developing and applying the knowledge needed to support children's wellbeing (see figure 4.1).

CHILD WELLBEING

- Social and Emotional Development
- Attachment and Caregiving Relationships
- Understanding Concerning Behaviors
- Risk and Resiliency
- Family Relationships and Culture
- Caregiver's Sphere of Influence

STRENGTH-BASED CAREGIVING

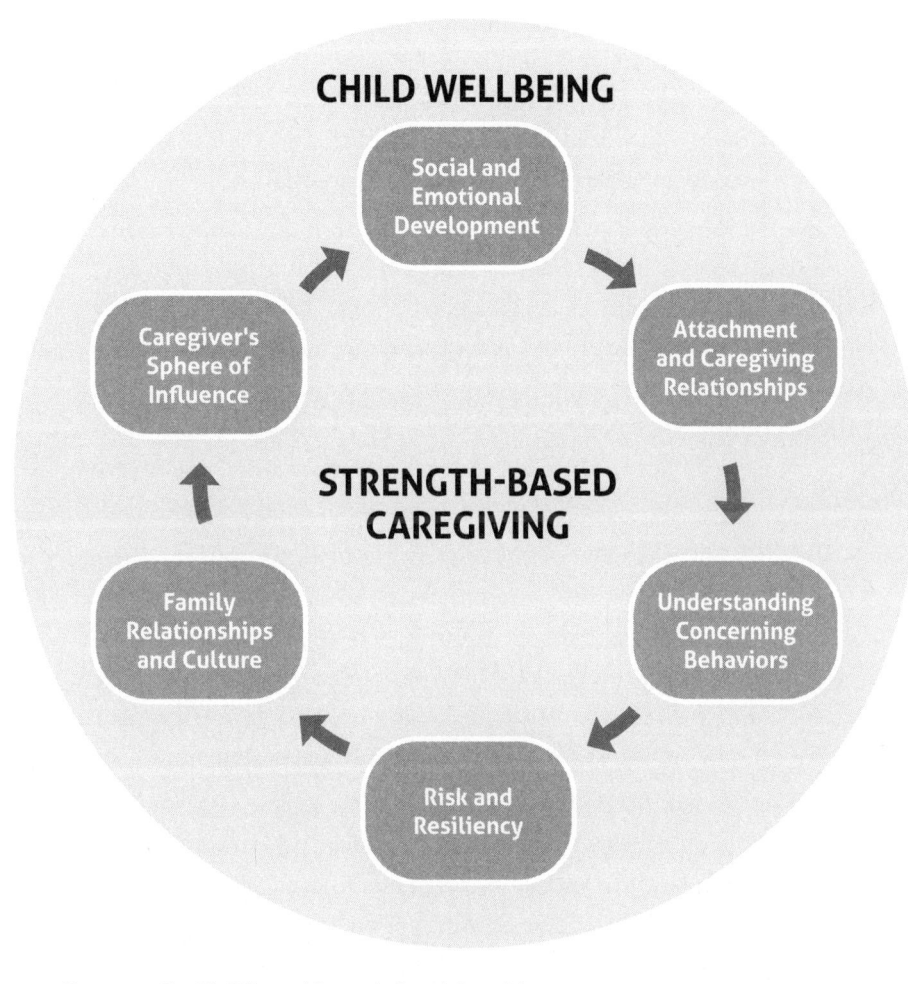

Figure 4.1. The Six Pillars of Strength-Based Caregiving

While each pillar is detailed in section 2 of the book, below are descriptions of each pillar. As you begin to adapt your strength-based professional practice, you will draw from multiple pillars as you engage in strength-based caregiving with children.

The first pillar, *Social and Emotional Development*, is key as children begin in infancy to develop their capacity for experiencing and regulating a broad range of emotions, form secure relationships, explore their environment, learn, and grow. Children acquire social skills that allow them to navigate their relationships with people and emotional skills to support them in understanding and interpreting their emotional experiences.

The second pillar, *Attachment and Caregiving Relationships*, builds on the first pillar—it is the bond that develops between caregivers and young children, which supports the development of both social and emotional skills in the classroom.

The third pillar, *Understanding Concerning Behaviors*, focuses on atypical behaviors that may be alarming to adults. Children with concerning behaviors may need a referral to a mental health professional.

The fourth pillar, *Risk and Resiliency*, refers to individual, relational, communal, and societal factors that impair healthy attachment or cognitive, language, physical, or social and emotional development. Risk factors place stress on a young child's development and thus affect how relationships are formed and how the brain is wired. Resiliency refers to individual and environmental protective factors, including health, mental health, nutrition, family supports, early care and education, and specialized services.

The fifth pillar, *Family Relationships and Culture*, acknowledges that a family is the first and most important relationship for a child. Families, community, and culture influence many aspects of the developing child, including how they form relationships, communicate their needs, go out into the world and come back, take risks, and respond to adversity and trauma. All other pillars are influenced by family and culture.

The sixth pillar, *Caregiver's Sphere of Influence*, refers to your role in a child's social and emotional wellbeing, which includes a strong knowledge of child development, the use of observation, and your own reflective practice to make ethical decisions about supporting young children. It involves understanding the many facets of social and emotional development and having the skills to address complex behavioral needs in the classroom. This pillar also includes accurately knowing when and where to secure supports for children who do not respond to developmentally appropriate guidance over time.

Together the Six Pillars build the foundation for a strength-based approach within responsive and dyadic caregiving. While each pillar is reviewed individually, they should be woven together in your practice as you think about young children and families.

Supporting Young Children through Strength-Based Approaches

The Six Pillars offer a way to frame your observations and questions to build wellbeing in young children. Here are questions we recommend asking when seeking to support children birth through age five and their families:

- *Pillar 1, Social and Emotional Development:* How is the child progressing along the developmental continuum of social and emotional competencies? How is the child communicating their needs to their caregivers? What additional information would be useful?
- *Pillar 2, Attachment and Caregiving Relationships:* What do I know and what do I observe about the dyadic relationship between the child, the family, and myself, the caregiver? How do I reflect and document the child's classroom social and emotional health? What additional information would be useful?
- *Pillar 3, Understanding Concerning Behaviors:* What collaborative community resources can I partner with to support the child and the family? What supports do I need in my professional practice to support the child? What additional information would be useful?
- *Pillar 4, Risk and Resiliency:* What do I know about the child's environment inside and outside of the program? What do I know about the child's history? What additional information would be useful?
- *Pillar 5, Family Relationships and Culture:* What do I know about the individual child, their community, and their culture? How can I leverage the family's cultural knowledge and strengths? What are the social and emotional resources and skills within their culture that the family can draw from? What additional information would be useful?
- *Pillar 6, Caregiver's Sphere of Influence:* What personal strengths can I draw from to support the child in my classroom? What will I do to support home-school connections and integrate services and supports into my classroom? What additional information would be useful?

While the Six Pillars are listed in order, you may work through the questions in any way that makes the most sense in a given situation. Though some questions will not apply in some cases, always review all Six Pillars to ensure you are focused on a strength-based approach. Consider

Ava in the theoretical story below; this vignette presents a scenario in which to consider how you might apply the questions from the Six Pillars.

> *A little over five months ago, Ava moved from another country and started attending your school. Prior to moving, Ava had attended a school close to her grandmother's house where they had walked together to school every day. To help with the transition to a new country, Ava's grandmother came with the family to help everyone settle into their new routines. Ava's grandmother returned home last week, and now Ava, her mother, and her father are adjusting to their new routine.*
>
> *Ava, who is three and a half, is dropped off late at school on a particularly busy morning. The classroom is full of activity as several new students started today. Ava tends to struggle with transitions from home into the classroom. While her caregivers and her parents have worked together to try to create a successful transition for Ava, it seems that her anxiety about separating from her parents is leading to an increased frequency of crying at drop-off. This behavior is very different from drop-off at her previous school before she moved.*
>
> *While her mother tries to leave, Ava clings to her leg while tears run down her cheeks. Ava's mother squats down at her level and tells her she will be back later. Ava's caregiver reaches around and holds her close as her mother leaves. Ava continues to silently cry, clinging to the caregiver's leg. After about fifteen minutes, the caregiver has had no success after having tried everything she knows to facilitate a successful transition.*

You can practice and grow your skills in supporting young children's wellbeing by applying the Six Pillars to Ava's story. Ask yourself, *How could I apply a strength-based approach to responsive caregiving in this scenario?*

Pillar 1, Social and Emotional Development: How is the child progressing along the developmental continuum of social and emotional competencies? How is the child communicating their needs to their caregivers? What additional information would be useful?

- Ava is developmentally on track across social, emotional, cognitive, language, and physical domains.
- Ava's family came from another country, and her English is rapidly developing.

- Her parents indicate that her vocabulary has grown, but she rarely speaks in class.
- When she speaks with others, she is shy.
- You think Ava seems to be developmentally on track for some emotional domains, but observing her emotional interactions when she spends so much of her day at your side is difficult to do.

Pillar 2, Attachment and Caregiving Relationships: What do I know and what do I observe about the dyadic relationship between the child, the family, and myself, the caregiver? How do I reflect and document the child's classroom social and emotional health? What additional information would be useful?

- Ava has a close, loving relationship with both her parents, although her dad only occasionally comes to school.
- She was especially close to her grandmother, who was her primary caregiver before she started child care, and she walked Ava to school after she entered care outside the home.
- As her caregiver, you find Ava to be sweet and loving, but you struggle to focus additional attention on her during the busiest time of the day.
- You now find yourself sometimes frustrated after having tried so many different approaches for the past five months with little success.
- Ava's struggles are especially evident during morning transitions.
- Ava is physical healthy and rarely absent.
- You feel bad that you experience a sense of relief on the few days Ava is absent from class.

Pillar 3, Understanding Concerning Behaviors: What collaborative community resources can I partner with to support the child and the family? What supports do I need in my professional practice to support the child? What additional information would be useful?

- As frustrated as you are, your heart breaks a little for Ava.
- While willing to talk about transition times, the family seems reluctant to address what might be the unmet need creating Ava's concerning behavior.
- The parents mention that Ava regularly has nightmares.
- You wonder what role the stress of Ava's recent move, separation from her grandmother, and establishment of new routines plays in her concerning behavior.

Pillar 4, Risk and Resiliency: What do you know about the child's environment inside/outside of the program? What do you know about the child's history? What additional information would be useful?

- Ava lives two miles from school, which is too far to walk.
- Her mother drops her off most days.
- In her previous school in her country of origin, there was a long transition period, and her grandmother would often walk Ava to school and then remain during that transition period, reading stories to Ava or listening to her plans for the day.
- During your parent conference with Ava's parents, they shared that they consciously decided to ask Ava's grandmother to no longer pick up or drop off Ava after they moved so they could create only one school routine, as Ava's grandmother would be returning to her home.
- It is important to Ava's parents that Ava learn to be independent.

Pillar 5, Family Relationships and Culture: What do I know about the individual child, their community, and their culture? How can I leverage the family's cultural knowledge and strengths? What are the social and emotional resources and skills within their culture that the family can draw from? What additional information would be useful?

- You know that Ava's family moved to the United States in the last year and that Grandma has recently gone back to her home.
- While the parents are bilingual, Ava previously spoke her primary language at home with Mom and Grandma, but her parents now both speak English with her at home to prepare her for school.
- Ava's mom has commented that Ava struggles whenever she is left in the care of others.
- You do not agree with letting Ava struggle.

Pillar 6, Caregiver's Sphere of Influence: What personal strengths can I draw from to support the child in my classroom? What will I do to support home-school connections and integrate services and supports into my classroom? What additional information would be useful?

- You continue reading articles and books to find an approach that will work with Ava.
- You want to tell Ava's parents that she appears unhappy in your class and that you worry about how her experiences will affect her future engagement in school.

- Your director has come to observe Ava during the morning transition and encourages you to work out Ava's difficulties yourself.
- This response leaves you feeling stressed, as you need both support and a direction to follow.
- You feel alone in this task of supporting Ava, as your director and the parents view Ava's struggle as a natural transition process to her new routine.
- You feel that your classroom environment is now emotionally unhealthy for Ava.

Ava's experiences highlight the complex interactions that take place in our classrooms every day. You know that Ava lives in a loving home with caring parents. You also feel deeply concerned about Ava's atypical behaviors and how they will affect her social and emotional development. You have some ideas about what might be contributing to Ava's continued distress in the program. You know that Ava's struggle cannot continue but are uncertain of what steps to take next.

In this chapter, we will reflect on each pillar and create a coordinated plan for Ava. Employing a strength-based approach, we will work to identify what is in our sphere of influence to support Ava in our program and what resources and experts we need to identify outside of our classroom setting. Keep Ava and her family in mind as you move through the book.

TABLE 4.1. REFLECTIONS ON THE SIX PILLARS

SIX PILLARS OF STRENGTH-BASED CAREGIVING	WHAT DO YOU KNOW ABOUT THE SIX PILLARS?	WHAT DO YOU STILL WANT TO LEARN ABOUT THE SIX PILLARS?	WHAT QUESTIONS DO YOU STILL HAVE ABOUT AVA?
Pillar 1: Social and Emotional Development			
Pillar 2: Attachment and Caregiving Relationships			

www.redleafpress.org/scm/4-1.pdf

Pillar 3: Understanding Concerning Behaviors			
Pillar 4: Risk and Resiliency			
Pillar 5: Family Relationships and Culture			
Pillar 6: Caregiver's Sphere of Influence			

Final Thoughts

The framework of the Six Pillars is designed to support us in taking a 360-degree view of what is happening in a young child's life to observe their development and behavior from many perspectives. This framework helps us develop the skills we need to provide strength-based caregiving. In a strength-based early learning environment, caregivers inherently believe that human beings have the capacity to learn, grow, and develop to their full potential, regardless of their age or ability. Responsive caregivers believe that the human spirit is resilient. Caregivers build on the individual child's strengths, desires, interests, talents, resiliency, and temperament.

A young child's mental health develops within the context of their family. Young children develop social skills, including a sense of self and self-identity, within their family culture. Families are guided by cultural beliefs and principles they in turn convey to their children through activities, behaviors, and attitudes. Knowing that families experience different dynamics, histories, and living situations, caregivers build on the strengths of each individual child and their family. Together caregivers and parents support one another in helping children to develop a sense of wellbeing and to reach their full potential.

A wide variety of services are available, both online and in person, to support both the child's development and the dyadic relationship. These supports include everything from screening and assessment to expert interventions that scaffold whole-child development. Knowledge of the continuum of supports and services will assist you in providing the best quality care you can to the children in your care. The support of other professionals, screenings, and services all help strengthen the safety net around children and their families. Based on the needs or complexity of the situation, professionals and support services can join caregivers in providing high-quality care to children and families.

Taking Action

What Caregivers Can Do

- Choose one pillar that is less familiar to you. Create a list of questions that you might want to answer to help you in using this particular pillar.
- Review the Six Pillars and their corresponding questions when a child demonstrates concerning or challenging behavior in your classroom.
- Reflect on the Six Pillars framework, making a list of areas of your personal strengths and areas for improving your caregiving practice.

Reflection and Application

- How might you use the Six Pillars in your practice?
- What additional skills do you need to support you in implementing the Six Pillars?
- How do you see the Six Pillars adding to best practices in your program?

SECTION 2

The Six Pillars

In this section, we dive deeper into the Six Pillars of responsive caregiving. Each chapter is designed to deepen your understanding of the pillar and the research that is the foundation for the information in each chapter.

- Chapter 5: Social and Emotional Development—understanding typical social and emotional development, which is the foundation of all strength-based caregiving
- Chapter 6: Attachment and Caregiving Relationships—understanding the dyadic relationship between you and each individual child in your care
- Chapter 7: Understanding Concerning Behaviors—understanding that children exhibit varying behaviors that may link to mental health disorders
- Chapter 8: Risk and Resiliency—understanding both risk and protective factors that impact a child's mental wellness
- Chapter 9: Family Relationships and Culture—understanding families and their cultures and identifying the multitude of approaches needed in culturally responsive practice
- Chapter 10: Caregiver's Sphere of Influence—understanding how you can support children's mental health and wellbeing and how to access services and supports

CHAPTER 5

Pillar One: Social and Emotional Development

Learning to deal with setbacks and maintaining the persistence and optimism necessary for childhood's long road to mastery are the real foundations of lasting self-esteem.
—Lillian Katz

Social and emotional development is essential for the growing child and their sense of wellbeing. It is among the most complex work that humans do. The ability to develop and navigate human emotions is a lifelong process. Social and emotional skills are best developed in relationships with others that allow children to freely explore and develop who they are in safe, secure, and nurturing environments that foster positive social and emotional skills and wellbeing. It is the back-and-forth, or serve-and-return, of human interaction that scaffolds social and emotional development. Curricular tools such as reading books or helping children learn problem-solving strategies are useful in teaching concepts about social and emotional development, but as we have shared throughout this book, the child's relationships with their primary caregivers lay the foundation for early brain development and social-emotional development. Secure, loving relationships with adults are foundational to healthy child wellbeing.

Social and emotional skills are not learned separately but rather are developed along with the other learning domains of cognitive, language, and physical development. Because learning is integrated, we know that acquiring social and emotional skills is a dynamic process. Each child develops a sense of self and wellbeing in their own way and in their own time. For example, some children easily acquire skills such as sharing or showing empathy, while other children, and sometimes even adults, have difficulty sharing and caring for others. As early childhood caregivers, we monitor how children develop and meet milestones in all areas of learning, including the child's ability to express themselves and interact with others in healthy ways. Promoting the competencies of social and emotional development in young children is one of the roles of quality care.

Understanding Child Wellbeing

In this chapter, we will focus on emotional wellbeing. Chapter 8 provides a closer look at children's unmet needs or traumatic experiences and their effect on mental health. As caregivers, we begin by understanding that wellbeing is a blend of social and emotional competencies and internal self-concepts (see tables 5.1 and 5.2 for a full list of competencies). Emotional wellbeing or wellness focuses on children's internal concepts of self, which include beliefs and feelings, such as, *I feel trust, and caregivers are trustworthy* and *I am respected, valued, protected, comforted, and loved.* Wellbeing is a complex state influenced by many factors that is achieved when children's basic social, emotional, cognitive, language, and physical needs are met.

Social and emotional wellness includes feelings that are highly individualized, which is why several children who experience the same event may feel and react differently. Healthy social and emotional development leads to children's strong sense of self and wellbeing. Wellbeing emerges in children who feel secure in their relationships with trusted, consistent, reliable adults. Respectful reciprocal relationships inside and outside the classroom foster children developing a positive concept of self.

We will examine each of the five components of social and emotional health in children (see figure 5.1). Each domain has its own structure that influences the social and emotional health of the child. All domains need to be supported for children to develop

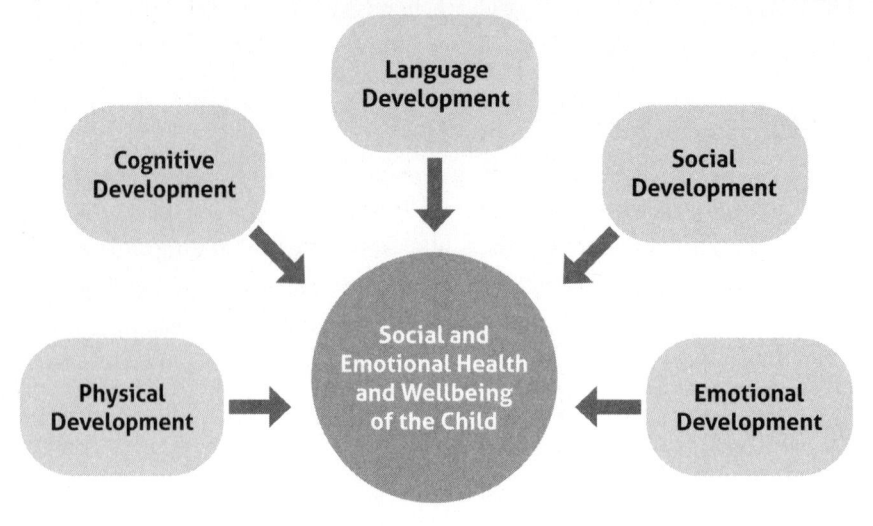

Figure 5.1. Social and Emotional Health of the Child

social and emotional health. As we look at the domains, we will begin by exploring how the domains interact, starting with physical development.

Physical Development

The physical development of children includes motor development, both gross and fine, along with perceptional development. Perceptional development describes the ability to perceive the world through the senses. This includes vision, hearing, smell, taste, and touch. Physical development follows a predictable pattern, moving from simple to complex and from large movement to small movement. As caregivers, we assess whether children are meeting their developmental milestones. Early care providers need to carefully document if they observe delays in a child's development and share their concerns with the child's parents. Referrals are typically made to pediatric or family practice physicians when children are not meeting milestones. Physicians will assess the child's development and make recommendations for support or early intervention.

Physical development is linked to child wellness through the active movement of the body. Physical activity for young children involves movement and play. There are strong correlations between children's self-directed activities, such as free play, and mental wellbeing. All elements of play contribute to mental health. We discussed the importance of play in chapter 1. We know that through play, children lay the foundation for self-control, cooperation, sharing, taking initiative, and imagination. Play fosters social interactions and boosts self-confidence as children learn to interact with others and read the social and emotional cues of peers and adults.

Other factors that affect physical wellbeing include the children's home and early care environments. Environmental impacts include access to adequate and nutritious foods, safe environments, shelter, sleep, and health care, including immunizations. Here are some examples of what safe environments can encompass:

- space that invites movement and exploration
- space free from toxins or environmental hazards
- space where adults treat children with respect
- space free of physical, social, or emotional threats (or inconsistency)
- community that is safe to navigate

Physical needs bridge home and school. Children's wellness and behavior are negatively affected when their basic needs for physical development are not met. Remember when evaluating a child's behavior to first determine whether their physical needs are being met. For example, if a child had a poor night's rest or is overly tired, then they are less able to focus or follow simple directions, so they may struggle with social and emotional regulation and interactions with others.

> These are some different types of physical needs:
>
> Body and hygiene: Children get enough sleep for their age; their sleep patterns are consistent; they have morning and bedtime routines; and they have hygiene habits such as bathing, toileting, and tooth care as part of their regular care.
>
> Medical and dental: Families have a medical home and a consistent doctor; children's growth and development are monitored through regular checkups; children go to the dentist and have healthy teeth; and allergies and other common childhood chronic conditions are addressed.
>
> Nutritional: Children are provided a healthy diet of balanced food groups based on family food preferences, and regular meals and snacks in appropriate serving sizes are provided both at home and in caregiving settings.
>
> Motor: Children are physically active, using both large- and small-motor muscle groups, and families and caregivers minimize sedentary activities such as watching TV, playing video games, and other forms of passive entertainment.

The American Academy of Pediatrics further offers recommendations on children's physical needs and wellness. Caregivers also need to understand that all body needs are defined within the cultural context of the family. Identifying and meeting the child's unmet physical needs is part of fostering healthy social and emotional development.

Cognitive Development

Cognitive development focuses on how children think and understand the world. From birth, children are actively taking in information and learning, thinking, and exploring the world around them. As children's cognition develops, they are able to mentally hold on to ideas and concepts such as following directions and understanding the meaning of class guidelines. They are better able to see themselves as separate from others, develop self-reflection skills, problem solve, anticipate next steps, and initiate social interactions.

In 1973 Jean Piaget (1896–1980) asserted that children construct their own learning as they explore and investigate the world through trial and error and play. Piaget theorized that physical skills, including motor and sensory exploration, help formulate children's early learning. He suggested that the development of children's thinking processes moves through four distinct stages of development: sensorimotor, preoperational reasoning, concrete preoperational reasoning, and formal operational reasoning stages. The first two stages align with children ages birth through five years.

Sensorimotor Stage (birth–2 years): In the first two years of life, young children primarily recognize the world around them based on their physical interactions and sensory exploration. During infancy, young children orient themselves to their environment and to their caregivers, so consistent and predictable routines, caregiving strategies, and environments are important for children's developing sense of safety and trust. In this stage of development, children build cognitive skills by physically manipulating themselves within their environment, which is typically done as they learn to crawl, walk, and run; feed themselves; and explore their world through play. Around nine months of age, infants begin to recognize object permanence, recognizing that an object that is no longer visible still actually exists. They are also learning about cause and effect, building memory and mental representations (see description below), and connecting experiences.

Preoperational Reasoning Stage (2–7 years): The ability to solve problems begins to develop during the sensorimotor stage (around 9 months). Children begin to use drawing and language to symbolically represent objects. They begin to solve problems by focusing on a single aspect of the problem at a time. They are learning to follow simple directions and enjoy engaging in play activities such as hide-and-seek, putting together wooden puzzles, and playing with soft blocks and toys.

Jerome Bruner (1915–2016) looked at cognitive development from another perspective, considering how children organize and represent their thinking. Bruner believed that from infancy to adulthood, we construct knowledge through three specific models (1985); the ages next to each stage represent when children first develop these cognitive skills.

Enactive Representation (0–1 year): Learning occurs through physical interaction (action-based). This is the foundation of the concept of learning by doing. Learning by doing empathizes experiential learning and engagement with the environment. From infants who explore objects to adults who engage in physical activity, our learning occurs through physical engagement and builds muscle memory. For example, we invoke muscle memory as we walk, run, or move our legs in a consistent pattern.

Iconic Representation (1–6 years): In this type of image-based learning, we create pictures or mental representations in our mind. For example, think about reading a book. Do you see the words or the images the words create? We learn to collect mental representations of like objects. For example, if I asked you to think about a dog, you would immediately conjure up your own unique image of a dog. This image or representation would be based on your overt or covert experiences with dogs. Through experiences and observations, we learn that there are different kinds of dogs and that they can be different sizes and have different features. You might have petted a dog and then gained a sense of what a dog's fur feels like or what a dog looks like when it barks or wags its tail. Collectively, these experiences and images form your unique mental representation of a dog, and might include feelings of happiness, joy, or excitement. Mental representations help us store and later recall information from our memory. This is also how viewing an image or drawing an object, or seeing, tasting, or holding a concrete object helps us learn new skills. This knowledge reminds us that early literacy needs to be built on children's mental representation of concepts rather than rote memorization, although exposure to and exploration of symbols is important.

Symbolic Representation (6 years onward): Our ability to use language (language-based learning) and its representative symbols (letters, numbers, or musical notes, for example) emerges as our cognitive process allows us to combine symbols to make meaning (such as a book or a musical score). Symbolic representation develops later in young children, because unlike a picture, symbols can be rearranged or changed in more than one combination. Symbolic representation skills are important as children learn more about spatial awareness and mathematical concepts.

Both Piaget and Bruner's theories offer examples of stages of cognitive development. These theories, along with Lev Vygotsky's (1896–1934), who spoke of scaffolded learning and socially constructed learning, form the foundation for many learning theories used today in education. Understanding that cognitive development can be viewed through different theoretical frameworks helps us to start to reflect on the many interpretations of how children develop. Acknowledging that there are many theoretical frameworks of child development helps us to embrace a strength-based approach to documenting children based on the interpretation of child development we use.

Language Development

Learning language is one of childhood's fundamental tasks. Beginning at birth, infants are ready to interact and communicate with others. They are busy watching, imitating, and learning the sounds and meanings of words and gestures. Every language has its own set of sounds, tones, and speech patterns. The more that children ages birth to three years hear language spoken in the form of social interactions, reading, and singing, the more the brain wires itself for language.

Language involves a give-and-take of words and gestures. This give-and-take, sometimes called serve and return, provides children with experiences to develop and strengthen their language skills. You can have conversations with infants who can't yet speak by mimicking their vocalizations or using self-talk to share what you're doing. For example, you might say, "I'm going to put on your shoes and socks so we can go outside and play." Self-talk allows children to make connections between spoken language and objects, gestures, and actions. For example, if you demonstrate waving and say the words, "Bye-bye," a child will begin to mimic the gesture and make cognitive connections between the words and the gesture. You might also scaffold a child's feelings when they are dysregulated by saying, "It looks like you are upset. I wonder how I can help you."

The sequence of learning language is universal. All children around the world learn language in the same sequence. First, receptive language is developed as babies listen to the language that surrounds them. The brain begins to wire connections from the sounds and tones to the language(s) heard. Their attentiveness and reactions to the voices and faces of familiar adults are their first steps toward acquiring spoken language.

Next, children begin developing expressive language by crying for food, warmth, physical comfort, and companionship. Cooing and babbling follow as children mature and begin making social and emotional connections with siblings, adults, and caregivers. Children typically speak their first recognizable words between ages ten and fourteen months. Vocabulary then quickly develops, and typically around the age of eighteen to twenty-four months, children begin forming two- to three-word sentences. Acquiring early expressive and receptive language skills are important milestones. If you observe children showing delays with language development, be sure to follow your employers' protocol for follow-up assessment and parent referrals.

Helping children make connections between feelings, interactions, and language can be fun. Learning social and emotional language begins early. Begin slowly introducing words and using simple sentences, such as, "Do you need help?" or "Are you feeling sad because Mama left for work?" The simple use of words and sentences helps children begin the process of connecting actions, feelings, and social and emotional words.

As toddlers become more autonomous and master new skills such as feeding themselves, meltdowns and tantrums are not uncommon. More often than not, young children are learning to use their words through trial and error. This process of learning to express themselves can cause frustration, and at times young children can become inconsolable. The more toddlers develop simple ways to express their needs and wants, the fewer tears and meltdowns you will see. Help toddlers build social and emotional language through reading, singing, and talking with them. Remember to introduce these activities when children are relaxed and the brain is in a calm state. Keep it simple, be patient, and encourage them as they develop these skills.

Children ages three to five years engage in more cooperative play and social interactions with peers and adults. They too are rapidly building their social and emotional skills and the required language to express their needs and wants. Building friendship skills, showing empathy, and caring for others is also part of this development. Find ways to integrate social and emotional skills and language in all areas of your day. The more you can integrate learning, the better children can make connections, build on prior knowledge, and strengthen their cognitive skills. Dramatic play areas are great places to help children expand language skills, along with flannel-board stories and puppet play. Caregivers model and foster the development of prosocial values such as empathy, caring, compassion, truth, justice, kindness, responsibility, honesty, and many others. Building language allows children to learn these prosocial skills.

Social Development

Social development encompasses how we interact with others, work to get our needs met, and express ourselves. Social development allows us to work in groups, express and regulate our emotions, and navigate a world based on interactions and relationships. Throughout our lives, we are influenced by the relationships that we develop with others. For our youngest children, these are relationships with parents, close family such as grandparents, friends, and care providers. Social development is founded upon secure attachments with caring adults. Your role as caregiver is important because you are one of the first individuals outside of the parents who cares for children. Children learn to care for others from those who first cared for them. From our earliest attachments, we begin to learn who is kind, caring, and responsive to our needs and who is not. The care you provide strengthens the child's neuropathways and positively wires the brain. Responsive caregivers help children form secure attachments and a sense of self that is worthy of love and attention.

Emotional Development

Emotional development helps us focus on developing, understanding, expressing, and navigating a wide range of human emotions. Since infants and very young children respond to touch and sensory stimulation, loving and nurturing care is vital to emotional development, which begins early when mothers kiss and cuddle with their newborn babies and say, "I love you." From infancy, children are learning about their emotions. Like adults, children's emotions are experienced and stored in the body as well as the brain. In fact, young children first feel their emotions as changes in their heartbeat, breathing, and other physical responses. Our emotions are housed in the limbic system of the brain, which is the brain's feeling part. The logical part of the brain is the frontal cortex, where we do our critical thinking and problem solving. Imagine that there is a trapdoor between the emotional and logical parts of our brain that closes off the logical part when emotions overwhelm us, so that all we can do in that state is feel. Children can often be overtaken or hijacked by their feelings, and when this happens, their logical brain is not open for problem solving. Learning to understand and regulate our feelings is a lifelong process.

To support emotional development in young children, we begin by modeling and then connecting our thoughts, behaviors, and emotions as we care for them. The congruency between the caregiver's facial expression, tone of voice, and handling of a child sends as much of a message as do spoken words. For example, when a child takes in cues that their caregiver is feeling frustrated, impatient, or distant with them, yet also wants to hold or cuddle them, the child becomes confused by the mixed messages.

Beginning in infancy, caregivers can help children develop emotional vocabulary and name their feelings. As caregivers, we begin with simple language to help children match feelings to primary emotions such as sadness, anger, and happiness, to name a few. We help children expand their emotional vocabulary by observing children's behavior, then vocalizing what we see. Over time and as children mature, we add complexity to the words to help children learn that feelings come in degrees. For example, we can feel mad, but also at the same time feel frustrated, upset, or annoyed, and so on: "I am so *excited* to read our story, yet a little *frustrated* that I cannot find the book." This is particularly important because we often just name one emotion we are feeling to the child, but we know we often feel more than one at once.

The skill of identifying our range of feelings takes time and practice. Find ways to integrate emotional development throughout the day and in all curricular activities. See chapter 11 and the QR codes for a list of classroom activities designed to support children's social and emotional wellness and literacy. Using emotionally complex language is another way to support young children in navigating the depth and breadth of their feelings. The more children learn about the range of human emotions and are able to articulate how they feel, the more skilled they will be at learning to regulate their emotions.

Emotional Wellness

Emotional wellness focuses on the child's internal concept of self. One of the tasks of childhood is for children to learn who they are in the world, develop a sense of self and self-identity. Self can be defined by knowing oneself, understanding one's emotions, wants, and needs. Self-identity can be defined as the process of coming to understand who we are in relationship to the groups to which we belong. Groups are the social relationships and roles we have within our family, classroom, community group, culture, and race, to name a few.

Developing self-identity is a dynamic process, and what young children experience in early childhood settings influences how they see themselves in the world. Our prosocial values, such as respect for others, compassion, and honesty, also strongly influence who we are in the world. We discussed prosocial values in chapter 1, examining how these values strongly influence our thoughts, opinions, and reactions to certain behaviors. But more importantly, these values influence our internal state of self and self-identity. The concept of self-awareness is connected to self and self-identity, which encompasses our likes and dislikes, our spatial awareness of where our body is in relation to others and the environment, and our ability to communicate our needs so they are met. These online activities provide classroom approaches and activities for fostering self-awareness and self-identity in young children.

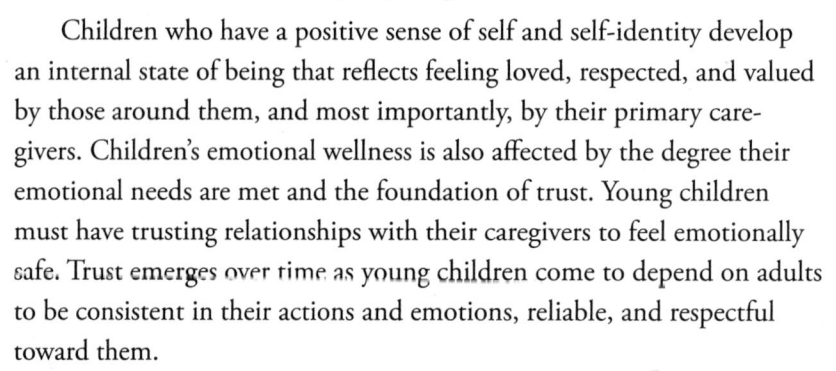

Children who have a positive sense of self and self-identity develop an internal state of being that reflects feeling loved, respected, and valued by those around them, and most importantly, by their primary caregivers. Children's emotional wellness is also affected by the degree their emotional needs are met and the foundation of trust. Young children must have trusting relationships with their caregivers to feel emotionally safe. Trust emerges over time as young children come to depend on adults to be consistent in their actions and emotions, reliable, and respectful toward them.

Children develop emotional wellness through direct interactions with other children and adults and through observation. Children watch and model what adults do and say to determine how to act and what meaning to assign to actions and words. Children's emotional wellness is adversely impacted when caregivers demonstrate inconsistency between actions and words, exhibit inconsistent emotions during the day, or exhibit signs of frustration, anger, or stress. We know that the vast majority of communication is nonverbal, and children unconsciously pick up on physical cues such as heartbeat, energy levels, distractedness, and other physical manifestations of caregivers' emotional states, which tell children that the environment is not emotionally safe. Emotionally unsafe or inconsistent environments cause a stress response in young children's brains, ratcheting up how the child reacts to stress in the future.

Social and Emotional Competencies

Beginning in infancy, children develop social and emotional skills along a continuum. As their social world expands from relationships with the nuclear family to extended family, other caring adults, and peers in child care, they develop and experience a wider range of emotions. We know too that secure attachments positively influence how children progress along the developmental continuum. With support and guidance from nurturing adults, children build on prior knowledge and skills as they move through different stages of social and emotional development. This begins in infancy, starting with the stages of responding to and exploring behaviors and growing into the stage of building and integrating behaviors. Infant and toddler social and emotional skills are the building blocks of preschool and kindergarten competencies. Although children develop social and emotional skills at their own pace, they typically progress in a similar fashion. The social and emotional competency areas for infants, toddlers, and preschool children are as follows:

Self and Self-Identity: Self and self-identity are formed as children learn to internalize themselves as separate, unique individuals. They learn about their bodies and realize they can navigate in and out of space or areas in a classroom or home environment. They learn that they have families that look and sound different from others. They learn that they have self-agency and can make choices. They learn to follow rules, play, build relationships, explore their environment, and be creative. They are learning to recognize and name emotions and feelings. Through a healthy sense of self and self-identity, children show empathy, compassion, and confidence, and build strong relationships with others.

Self-Regulation: The ability to self-regulate develops over time and is based on secure attachments. Learning to self-regulate is influenced by many developmental and environmental factors. As children ages eighteen to twenty-four months learn to be more independent, they can become easily frustrated. Their language skills are still developing, so they have limited ability to articulate their needs and wants. Young children can quickly become tired or overstimulated, causing poor self-regulation. They are easily frustrated when caregivers place restrictions on what they can and cannot do, even though restrictions such as not hitting or biting are primarily for their safety and the safety of others. Children become better able to regulate their emotions and actions through maturation, clear reminders of class expectations, and improved communication skills. Guidance and patience from caregivers are important during these years while children are learning to identify and manage a wide range of emotions. Learning to regulate identified emotions also goes through stages of development, from self-soothing to later self-regulation. Learning to focus and attend to activities, control impulses, and improve communication skills will help the child's ability to self-regulate.

Social and Cultural Awareness and Respect: As children develop a sense of self and self-identity, they are also learning to see themselves within the larger context of a social community and culture. Adults who model and foster responsive, caring, and trustworthy relationships provide a foundation for social and emotional development. Caregivers who integrate cultural awareness into the environment help children deepen their connections to family and broaden their self-understanding. Children are also profoundly influenced by the beliefs and values that classmates bring to the early learning environment. Developing skills of empathy, respect, and social awareness of diverse cultures and backgrounds is important for young children.

Relational Skills: For young children, developing relationships begins with their primary caregivers and later extends to their larger family, program or school, and community. As a child's network of relationships widens, their social and emotional skills also grow. Children must draw upon prior social and emotional knowledge and skills to learn how to successfully navigate and build relationships with adults and peers. Like other social and emotional skills, we know that relationship skills develop over time. Infants and toddlers form secure attachments with caregivers while also actively observing other children around them. Although infants and toddlers play independently, they learn about caring, empathy, and responsive social interactions by watching caregivers interact with peers. Early relationship skills are the foundation for later social and emotional development during the preschool and kindergarten years.

Infant and Toddler Competencies

In infants and toddlers, social and emotional competencies are founded upon respectful reciprocal relationships with caregivers who are responsive to young children's needs. Responsive caregiving demonstrates that children can trust adults to read their cues and meet their needs. In chapter 6, we review the importance of extending attachment from the home environment into the early childhood setting and consider your role as caregiver in this process. The following developmental competencies provide an overview of important skills and strategies caregivers can use to support young children. They are not a screening or assessment tool to determine whether a child is developmentally on track, but rather the skills that help children form a healthy sense of wellbeing.

TABLE 5.1. SOCIAL AND EMOTIONAL COMPETENCIES IN INFANTS AND TODDLERS

TOPIC	INFANTS/TODDLERS	CAREGIVERS
Self and Self-Identify	A growing awareness of one's body and how it works	Responding to infant and toddler cues in a timely fashion, building on the foundation of trust in adult
	An increasing awareness of the environment around oneself	Creating a balance of novelty (new ideas and activities to explore) and familiarity (routines and patterns of engagement that support children in feeling engaged and secure)
	A growing interest and ability to navigate the environment	Gradually providing more opportunities for young children to make choices
	A developing understanding of one's own and others' emotions	Being comfortable with all young children's emotions and providing supportive environments for young children to express their emotions
Self-Regulation	The developing ability to self-regulate by tuning out external stimuli	For infants, providing environments that allow them to self-regulate sleep and awake times; for toddlers, balancing the environment and scaffolding transitions between active and quiet times

PILLAR ONE: SOCIAL AND EMOTIONAL DEVELOPMENT

	An emerging awareness of boundaries and expectations	Supporting infants as they transition from biological schedules to routines; providing toddlers with simple expectations for classroom engagement and opportunities to practice expectations in a supportive environment
	The growing ability to help themselves or others in daily activities	Supporting infants as they communicate their needs for care (food, sleep, rest); supporting toddlers in scaffolding the beginning of self-help skills
Social Awareness	A growing sense that self is respected and valued by others	Asking infants for permission before moving them; offering choices to toddlers; encouraging children to try doing things on their own
	Building emotional connections with others and learning to respond to their emotional cues	Using language to explain the emotions of others; identifying ways to create emotional supports for them
	A developing awareness of being respected for who they are in the context of their family, program, school, and community	Offering choices to young children by working with families to identify culturally respectful ways of caregiving, such as feeding, toileting, sleeping, bathing, and clothing
Cultural Awareness and Respect	An emerging awareness and understanding that family routines, foods, and settings are different than their own	Creating connections between families to create shared experiences between children and adults
	Interest and enjoyment in new experiences different than home	Engaging and supporting new experiences for infants and toddlers
	A curiosity about people who are different than themselves	Responding to children's questions and observations about the world around them with ease; reflecting on culture though children's interests and experiences in their local community

Relational Skills	An emerging engagement in serve-and-return behavior or reciprocal exchanges in relationship with others	Creating serve-and-return engagement within the dyad; engaging in individual and sustained responses between you and a single child
	Engagement with others beyond primary caregivers; an increasing interest in new people	Helping children engage with others, both adults and children in the classroom and school community
	Learning to express emotions, increasing awareness of one's own and others' feelings, and learning to relate to others through empathy and caring	For infants, supporting, acknowledging, and addressing their emotional expressions in a timely manner; for toddlers, helping them learn to express emotions to create productive interactions

Preschool Competencies

As children enter the preschool years, their physical development reaches new milestones. Preschool children's awareness extends beyond their earlier focus on immediate experiences to an increasing awareness of the larger community. In these stages of development, young children begin to build on their emerging competencies in social and emotional development. While social and emotional competencies are sequential, you might notice that a child is still developing earlier competencies or experiencing social or emotional regression in times of stress.

TABLE 5.2. SOCIAL AND EMOTIONAL COMPETENCIES IN PRESCHOOLERS

TOPIC	PRESCHOOLERS	CAREGIVERS
Self and Self-Identity	An increasing sense of self and self-awareness	Scaffolding children's emotional vocabularies and emotions
	Continued development of likes and dislikes and offer opinions about choices and/or preferences	Demonstrating through interactions how to make choices or express preferences; offering supportive explanations when choices cannot be accommodated

Self-Regulation	A growing understanding of emotions and connecting them to words	Understanding that children have complex and overlapping emotions and that every child responds uniquely
	A growing ability to avoid harming others or materials when expressing themselves	Helping children talk out their emotions; once calm, reflecting on choices; understanding that this is an ongoing developmental process with lots of repetition
	Developing understanding of the importance of routines, boundaries, and classroom norms; exploring limits through trial and error	Creating spaces where classroom routines, boundaries, and norms are consistent, intentional, and flexible to meet all developmental needs.
	An ability to make choices and share the importance of choice	Supporting children by creating opportunities for them to make choices and share discoveries
Social Awareness	A developing sense of their right to be seen for their potential and for their abilities to be respected	Developing a positive emotional climate in the classroom where kindness is given and received between adults and children
	Developing compassionate responses to and empathy for the emotions of others	Supporting children in understanding and being comfortable with the full emotional spectrum, from joy to distress; being comfortable with all emotions displayed in the classroom
	Developing language and communication skills that allow them to engage each other	Scaffolding children in understanding intentions, asking questions, planning, negotiating, and reasoning with each other
Cultural Awareness and Respect	Learning to respect similarities and differences between different people and making connections to those in their classroom community.	Having inclusive classroom practices that invite all children's voices and perspectives; giving all children ownership of their classroom community by reflecting their cultural norms and languages
	The growing ability to understand another's point of view or experience	Supporting the development of empathy by helping children connect to how others might feel

	Showing a growing awareness of others' rights and responding respectfully	Supporting classroom expectations and connecting expectations to each child's rights in the classroom
	A growing sensitivity to the similarities and differences in others regarding language, culture, race, family, and gender expression	Scaffolding positive communication and interactions between and among peers; building cultural understanding through a wide variety of diverse books and materials
Relational Skills	A growing capacity to engage in sustained play and interactions with children and adults	Providing extended blocks of unscheduled time for children to independently engage with each other; scaffolding supports for children who have difficulty sustaining play with others
	Developing and sustaining friendships	Supporting children in engagement by helping them manage conflict and serve-and-return engagement
	The emergence of communication through words rather than actions across emotional responses and learning to seek support when needed	Supporting children in developing complex emotional vocabularies and connecting vocabulary to feelings; being open and accessible to children's requests for social and emotional supports when they engage with others

Short and Long-Term Goals of Caregiving

As we look at children's social and emotional development and how children learn to identify and regulate their emotions, we must also look at the short- and long-term goals of parenting and caregiving. It is important to recognize that cultural values influence parents' short- and long-term goals for their children, along with the prosocial values we identified earlier, including character traits such as honesty, trustworthiness, reliability, and kindness. One of the short- and long-term goals most adults have for children is that they will grow to be responsible, caring adults who show empathy and love for others. Often adults want children to care about the environment, show respect for others, and value social justice.

Many times adults try to manage children's behavior through short-term rewards such as food, prizes, stickers, and so on, or through punishments such as time-outs. Sometimes well-intended adults hover over children, not allowing them to take reasonable or age-appropriate risks or not supporting their natural curiosity and desire to explore their environment. We also see parents who do things for the parents' gain rather than for the child's benefit, those who push children beyond what is age appropriate, demanding unrealistic or unachievable goals that set the child up for stress and failure.

Long-term goals involve modeling and instilling values such as wonder, curiosity, a love of learning, resiliency, and self-discipline. Long-term goals help the child develop a strong sense of self, with confidence in their own abilities and a desire to take initiative. Long-term goals focus on the bigger picture and help children discover their sense of self and self-identity: who they are in the world, their gifts and talents, and how they can contribute to the wellbeing of society.

Final Thoughts

Strength-based early learning environments promote the developing social and emotional skills that are essential to a child's mental health and wellbeing. As a responsive caregiver, you play an important role in how children develop these skills. The more you incorporate social and emotional interactions and skills into your everyday activities, the more children will internalize the values of empathy, caring, compassion, patience, and love. As we look at the range of human emotions, keep in mind the short- and long-term goals of behaviors you support in your early learning environment and how your strength-based practices can increase children's sense of wellbeing. Learning social and emotional skills aligns with other forms of a child's development and builds healthy relationships with both adults and peers. Lastly, remember that social and emotional development takes time. Skills such as learning to share are never fully mastered, and even as adults we need to continue to deepen our compassion, empathy, and love for others. The following are strength-based practices that will help you promote social and emotional development in young children:

- Respond to children's needs in a consistent and predictable manner.
- Provide three to five classroom rules that are simple and easy for children to follow.
- Provide opportunities for children to learn about social and emotional skills through stories and songs.

- Personalize the names of characters in stories or songs to include the names of the children in your classroom.
- Respond to children with empathy when they fall or get hurt, and encourage empathy in the classroom by saying, "Oh, that must hurt! Who will help me care for Juan?"
- Read stories about and share pictures of children demonstrating a range of emotions.
- Repeatedly use children's names when conversing with them.
- Express interest and excitement in children's explorations and newly developing skills.
- Find time to interact with and show enthusiasm for each child, helping them feel special and loved.
- Smile and take time to look at and interact with children at their eye level.
- Demonstrate a positive attitude toward parents and children.
- Use positive and encouraging language as you support and interact with parents and children.

Taking Action

What Caregivers Can Do

- Integrate social and emotional development throughout the classroom's daily schedule.
- Research songs or stories to add to your personal library that enhance social and emotional development.
- Develop strength-based strategies to promote children's social and emotional development.

Reflection and Application

- What long-term goals can I help parents and children develop?
- What supportive and encouraging language can I use to support parents and children?
- What strategies can I incorporate to support children who are struggling to regulate their emotions?
- What social and emotional trainings can I take to build my skills as a caregiver?

CHAPTER 6

Pillar Two: Attachment and Caregiving Relationships

School is not a place for anonymous users, rather it is a place where people live a portion of their life together.
—Paola Strozzi

We believe that responsive caregivers want the children in their early childhood classrooms to thrive and reach their full potential, and we know that relationships are the foundation of mental health and wellbeing. Building strong, respectful reciprocal relationships begins early, shaping future relationships. When young children are cared for in a loving, nurturing, and responsive way, they develop close, secure relationships and attachment to the caring, loving adults who provide their early care. As children grow and develop, our hope is that their connections and attachment deepen. Forming attachments and secure relationships is biologically necessary for developing children's health and wellbeing.

Early learning settings are wonderful places for children to learn and practice social and emotional skills. Forming emotional connections with each child in your care allows you to foster the emotional supports children need to learn, grow, and develop social and emotional skills. Caregivers need to consider not only their own emotional health (chapter 3) but the overall wellbeing of the classroom. Wellbeing in the classroom focuses on emotional regulation and communication between and among members of the classroom community. Building a classroom where young children and their caregivers thrive requires careful consideration of all relationships among adults and children to support everyone's emotional health and wellness. In this chapter, we will explore strength-based practices to promote self-regulation in young children and look closer at attachment and how it influences mental health and wellbeing.

The Foundation: Attachment

Forming secure relationships and attachments is one of the primary tasks of childhood. The relationships we form throughout life deeply influence our sense of wellbeing and mental health, and secure attachments with caring adults form a protective factor around a child in the face of adversity. We talk more about protective factors and their influence on the child's wellbeing in chapter 8. In *secure attachment*, the child builds a deep, long-lasting dyadic connection to their primary adult caregiver or caregivers, which typically includes biological parent(s) but can also include a teacher or other primary caregiver. Similar to secure attachment, a *secure relationship* is based on a stable, trusting, and consistent caregiver. A secure attachment is a more profound, more intrinsic connection between adult and child. A relationship can exist without attachment, *but* attachment cannot exist without a relationship. The stronger the stability, security, trust, and love between adult and child, the more secure the attachment. Early attachments to primary caregivers—parents as well as care providers—form the basis of a child's feelings of security and their capacity to form trusting relationships later in life. Secure attachments and feelings of safety, trust, respect, and being valued are essential to a child's ability to understand and regulate their emotions.

In high-quality early learning environments, responsive caregivers form secure relationships with children while strengthening attachment between themselves and each child. Research demonstrates a strong correlation between children's secure attachment and their emotional wellbeing and mental health. Although children can form more than one secure attachment, parents are the primary source of security for young children. Beginning in the 1950s, researchers such as Harry Harlow (1905–81), John Bowlby (1907–90), and Mary Ainsworth (1913–99) emphasized the importance of the parent-child relationship. They explored how infants' behavior changed when they were exposed to strangers and separated from their parents. Ainsworth observed that infants varied in their degree of security based on the type of attachment they had with their primary caregiver. From this body of knowledge, we see how children's response to their primary caregivers varies based on the degree of attachment they have formed.

Attachment is recognized as a continuum from secure attachment to avoidant attachment, including resistant/ambivalent attachment and disorganized attachment. This final form of attachment is rarely seen. Securely attached children demonstrate contentment and confidence in the presence of their parents or primary caregivers. They freely explore, demonstrate flexibility and resilience to changes in their environment, and respond to other children and adults with curiosity and warmth. They sense that the world is a safe and trusting place. Here are some signs caregivers will observe in securely attached infants, toddlers, and preschool children:

Infants and Toddlers

- They show delight by smiling, cooing, or wiggling their arms and legs when they see their parents and familiar adults.
- They relax and respond with ease when being held or fed.
- They gaze into the eyes of familiar adults.
- They sit and cuddle with familiar adults.
- They make efforts to communicate through sounds and gestures.
- They smile, giggle, and show joyful enthusiasm.
- They engage in reciprocal play with adults.
- They observe and show concern through facial expressions and crying.
- They play independently and observe other children nearby.
- They can be soothed or comforted by familiar adults.
- They explore and show curiosity in new things.
- They wave hello and good-bye.

Preschool Children

- They demonstrate initiative and imagination.

- They demonstrate willingness to follow simple directions.
- They seek to explore and ask adults for assistance.
- They independently and cooperatively play with peers.
- They show autonomy.
- They try new things.
- They build friendships.
- They are self-directed in their learning.
- They show growing ability to self-regulate.

As children develop from birth to age five, they gain the ability to differentiate between various attachment figures such as parents, professional caregivers, and others. As children mature, they form additional relationships with other important figures such as grandparents, siblings, friends, and extended family members. Each new relationship provides opportunities for children to emotionally grow and expand their social and emotional skills. This coincides with the developing brain and its ability to form mental representations, which are stored in the brain as mental pictures and collections of thoughts, impressions, experiences, and features that represent an idea, person, or concept. Children in the first few years of life are constantly developing and expanding thousands of mental representations, and some of the most important are those of their primary attachment figures. Each demonstration and experience of care, comfort, and love influences their mental representation of their primary attachment figure.

Around the end of year three, children begin developing more complex social and emotional skills, including a sense of self and self-identity. Secure attachment in the first three years allows children to make and sustain friendships and later form close, intimate relationships. The maturation of cognitive and social and emotional skills allows young children to move beyond just reacting to the attached figure to actively engaging in the caregiver partnership. Developing children are able to separate their own needs from the needs of others, allowing them to recognize, anticipate, acknowledge, and feel empathy for attachment figures, caregivers, and later peers. Young children who have developed a secure attachment with their parents sometimes find it difficult to separate from them. We see this in our early care centers when children exhibit separation anxiety. This is a natural response when young children have to say goodbye to their loved one. Responsive caregivers understand this and make efforts to help children feel safe, secure, and cared for as they learn to trust and form secure relationships with their caregivers.

Understanding Wellbeing in the Early Childhood Classroom

How do we work toward healthy classrooms and respectful reciprocal relationships? We move back to the primary unit of attachment: the child-adult dyad. Healthy classrooms include early childhood caregivers who nurture individual relationships with each child. Relational work happens in the child-caregiver dyad (one child, one caregiver). This dyadic relationship looks and feels different from the relationship with the classroom community, as it is focused on spending time in serve-and-return interactions.

Dyadic relationships often focus on the nonverbal exchange of emotional cues. Think of the exchange between adult and infant when playing peek-a-boo—the child and adult go back and forth looking at each other, sending and receiving information to and from each other in a mutual exchange.

> *The baby looks at the caregiver, opening eyes wide as the baby views the caregiver.*
>
> *"Peek-a-boo," calls the caregiver in a singsong voice with a big smile as she opens her hands and uncovers her eyes.*
>
> *Laughter follows from the baby as she focuses on the caregiver's face and returns the smile. Her face is animated; feet and arms wiggle.*

This exchange demonstrates both attunement between the child and the caregiver and serve-and-return behavior. In older children, serve-and-return behavior includes verbal exchanges of ideas as well as nonverbal cues. Dyadic relationships are founded upon secure, attached relationships between children and caregivers that demonstrate both serve and return and attunement to each other's emotions.

Strength-based early learning prioritizes spending time with each individual child. We form attachment and trust by acknowledging children's experiences and views as serious and meaningful, and understand that listening to children is fundamentally connected to their sense of self-esteem and, in turn, their wellbeing. Listening attentively to children is different than talking to or at children. Discussions that are navigational, such as "Let's come to the rug" or "It's time to put on our coats and line up," are not serve-and-return exchanges of ideas. Listening requires us to respond to children by exchanging ideas in ways that are meaningful to their stage of development. Authentic listening considers the emotions of the child. We follow the child's lead in their readiness to speak. Interrupting a child's work or play to ask a question is also not authentic listening because it is not part of the respectful reciprocal relationship cycle. Authentic listening includes allowing a child to approach you for an ongoing exchange or sitting with a child or children and waiting for them to come to a natural stopping point to engage in a conversation.

Caregivers use strength-based language that is encouraging and promotes social and emotional competence by acknowledging and building on the child's skills. Approach 1: Using Encouraging Words (page 154) provides examples of a strength-based approach. Chapter 9 and tables 9.1 and 9.2 will help you with strength-based language in the classroom. Caregivers can start strength-based conversations with children by talking about things they have noticed or observed that are unique to each child.

Emotional Regulation in the Classroom

Supporting children's growth in all areas of development—cognitive, linguistic, physical, and especially social and emotional—requires us to be and act in many ways simultaneously. We model emotional complexity by not only helping children share their words but also by making our emotions visible when we communicate and helping children develop a vocabulary of emotional language that connects feelings to words.

Strength-based practices for caregivers that scaffold young children's social and emotional development may include the following competencies:

- the ability to name simple and complex emotions that we ourselves feel in our everyday practice
- the ability to self-regulate
- the ability to be emotionally present, prepared, and available for the work
- the ability to understand the points of view of others, such as parents, caregivers, and children
- the ability to understand the feelings of others and place ourselves in their experiences

- with older children, the ability to understand the impact of unkind words and criticism on the emotional wellness of another person, classroom, or program
- the ability to act with kindness and compassion
- the ability to support both simple and complex emotions, to be comfortable with big emotions, and to scaffold children in addressing those feelings in productive ways
- the ability to support children's self-regulation by scaffolding feelings, offering opportunities to practice, and maintaining developmentally appropriate expectations
- the ability to authentically listen, interpret, and reflect back emotions
- the ability to interpret children's unmet needs in ways that result in productive actions or behaviors, and to recognize that concerning behavior is the outward sign of an unmet need
- the ability to work with others, using healthy communication practices in constructive ways when addressing negative feelings about another person, classroom, or program
- the ability to recognize kindness and compassion, and acknowledge its presence in children and adults

Identifying, regulating, and expressing emotions and providing words for feelings is one of the primary educational supports that caregivers offer young children. The ability to name emotions and make a connection between *what we feel* and *how we think* is foundational to making connections between emotional and cognitive development. The ability to control emotions, thoughts, and actions is the basis of self-regulation. For example, when a child can recognize what they feel and act, they come to a caregiver to ask for help when a toy is taken by another child rather than hitting the other child or taking a toy back. We often hear early childhood caregivers say, "Use your words." This can be difficult for children who are still learning to connect feelings, words, and problem solving together. Consider the following sequence instead. First, validate the child's feelings: "I can see that you are frustrated because your block tower was knocked over." Next, reassure the child to help them begin to regulate their emotions. This may take the form of breathing together or acknowledging the hurt behind the feelings. Then ask, "What do you need?," recognizing that the child might not have the emotional vocabulary to clearly articulate what they need next. Finally, offer suggestions for next steps. Pause between each question to allow time for processing, especially when a child is emotionally dysregulated. You could ask questions such as, "Do you want to rebuild?" or "Do you want to play something else?" This is a teachable moment, but remember too that children learn best once they have reregulated and the brain is in a relaxed state. This is an example of a caregiver helping the child make connections between their thinking and their feelings.

Our emotions as caregivers are just as complex as the children's, and we must also identify, regulate, and express our own emotions. We often function as the emotional regulators of the early childhood classroom; our energy and tone set the mood for the day. Therefore, we must be aware of our own emotional states to be prepared to lead the emotional health of our classrooms. Reflective practice is important because it provides us space to understand, assign, and process our emotions as we reflect on our work with children. We must attend to our own emotional vocabulary, remembering to use both simple and complex words when describing our feelings. Further, it is important for both us and the children to combine emotional descriptors, acknowledging that emotions are not singular, but complicated and interwoven. When we share a welcoming statement such as, "I am excited to start our day and am sad that one of our friends is absent and will miss our trip to the park," we acknowledge and model the complexity of our feelings.

Empathy and compassion are developed over time. The developmental stages of these skills follow the development of cognitive and physical skills. Empathy and compassion begin with secure attachment and loving relationships in the first years of life and continue into toddlerhood as children begin tracking, understanding, and responding to the emotions of others. Responding to other children can be hard work. Handing back a toy they want or hugging someone who is crying shows that children are developing the foundations of compassion and empathy. As children start their preschool years, they begin to name emotions in others, for example, when Charlie exclaims, "Abdi is excited that they have a new puppy," or Katra shares, "Ethan is frustrated that his tower keeps falling over." As adults, our concern and empathy for others shows in many ways both in the classroom and in our program community. We support children by asking open-ended questions that build on their observations.

Caregiver: "Ethan, Katra noticed that you were frustrated because your block tower keeps falling over. What have you tried?"

Ethan: "I tried everything, and it just won't work!"

Caregiver: "Would you like some help?"

Ethan: "Um, okay."

Caregiver: "At gathering time, how might you ask our friends for ideas to help with your building challenge?"

Ethan: "I will tell them about my idea to build a ramp to make my cars go fast."

Caregiver: "Let's see what our friends suggest."

The dialogue between Ethan and his caregiver highlights the feelings that children have when engaged in playful learning in the classroom. While not using specific words to describe feelings, the conversation shows that there are many members of Ethan's classroom community who care for him and are willing to support him in brainstorming a solution to his problem. We work to scaffold conversations in the classroom as the caregiver did with Katra and Ethan.

When we consider social and emotional development and appropriate practice, we must recognize that children are just learning these skills, so their application will be imperfect. As caregivers, we ourselves are still working on these skills too—we spend our whole lives mastering this skill set. Social and emotional wellness is a lifelong practice and one area that we can keep developing over time. Therefore, we want to be especially generous and understanding of young children's struggles just as we are generous and self-compassionate toward ourselves. Children's brains are building connections in their early years, so appropriate practices in scaffolding social and emotional development take this into account by acknowledging that these skills are emerging. In our own lives as adults, we may be breaking old habits and practicing new skills, meaning we are building new connections in our brains.

Supporting Emotionally Healthy Classrooms

In strength-based classrooms, we need to model healthy interactions by actively promoting a positive learning community and setting aside our negative behaviors. We build positive emotional climates for children through our own adult interactions. Early childhood settings become negative spaces when adults gossip and make assumptions about others, which breaks the fabric of a positive collective community and indicates that we are not acting with compassion or showing empathy, kindness, and respect to others. Rather, we work to do the following:

- assume positive intentions
- ask for clarification when unsure of colleagues' meanings
- refrain from speaking about others in negative ways

The social and emotional health of children in the classroom is affected by our ideas about children and their capabilities. How we see children has a great influence on our work. When we see children as capable, we enter into a relationship in which we value children and their ideas and consider them co-constructors of our classroom life. Our words, thoughts, and actions are outward demonstrations of our values. If our actions demonstrate our values in our work with children, then those values become the seeds that help grow both our community and the next generation.

How we view children stems in part from our own childhoods and the messages we received while growing up. For example, many caregivers feel that they are not good at teaching a particular subject, like art. Art is an experimentation with materials to create something. Process art is the experience of creating art, and there is no right or wrong result. Product art is an artistic creation that others can recognize. How we view art (product or process) is based on our own experiences and the messages we received from adults during childhood. When we think about messages from childhood, we see where some of our ideas about art came from. Beliefs about art is just one example of how childhood messages influence adult perceptions. Therefore, reflecting on the origins of our beliefs and values about children's capabilities is important.

When we view the classroom as a place where we exercise control, entering into reciprocal relationships is difficult. When we lead every aspect of the day, we create a power structure that places the voice of the caregiver over the voices of children, which creates an imbalance in the classroom. This leads to high levels of stress in the caregiver, which likewise increases children's stress levels. When we utilize our voice too often in our work with children, the rich exchange of dialogue and the formulation of ideas is impaired. In contrast, sharing choices and making decisions with children develops a shared leadership to address power structures in the classroom. This partnership supports caregivers and children to co-construct their classroom curriculum based on emerging interests. You may worry that inviting children into shared leadership of the classroom may invite chaos; however, children who share leadership in the classroom instead demonstrate competence, and the classroom becomes more self-managing. Shared leadership between children and caregivers actually supports developing children's sense of self, self-awareness, self-esteem, and self-confidence. Shared leadership scaffolds caregiver-child relationships that model the caregiver's trust in the children. If children are always turning back to the caregiver to check for agreement, even while they are independently performing different activities, secure relationships won't form. The caregiver becomes the authoritarian figure in the classroom, leading and thus controlling all elements of the classroom community.

In a classroom where children share decision-making, they engage in sustained individual and small-group work on their own. When children demonstrate an unmet need in this environment, caregivers shift to working with the individual child. No longer do you need to address the group as a whole to maintain order and control when one child presents concerning behavior; you can instead walk over to that child and, based on a relationship of mutual respect, work with them one-on-one. The individual, deeply personal relationships we develop with children allow us to have authentic conversations. Successfully resolving conflicts in the classroom creates healing for both child and caregiver, reducing stress levels in each.

Taking Our Emotional Temperature

In strength-based early learning, we prepare for our classroom by preparing ourselves. Just like a thermometer, our emotions can run from cool to hot. Are there certain times during the day when you feel frustrated? One way you can check how hot or cool your emotions feel during the day is to create a timeline and check in at various times to take your emotional temperature. See the example of a timeline in figure 6.1 and adjust as appropriate for your schedule. Be sure to include transition, outdoor time, activity, meal, and other scheduled activities, and any times that tend to create emotional triggers.

Understanding our emotional temperature allows us to know when during the day we tend to be more or less resilient to what is happening in our classrooms. This knowledge can help us choose to remain calm. For example, if you know that afternoon snack is a stressful time for you, you can make sure your co-teacher supports you at that time, or make sure you are focused only on snack. You can also consider what might be causing that stress and what you can do to reduce or eliminate it.

Part of being emotionally present is the ability to take your classroom's emotional temperature. Caregivers are not the only ones affecting the room's emotional climate. Children come into the space with their own feelings and emotional preparedness—or not—for their day. We feel the emotional climate rise, fall, or remain steady during different times of the day. While emotionally regulating our classrooms, we need to pay attention to markers such as activity and noise levels. These markers indicate children's level of self-regulation. When our classrooms begin to run too hot, we know that children are beginning to dysregulate and we need to modify our approach. Caregivers can use strength-based language to help regulate their classrooms.

Markers Indicating the Emotional Regulation of the Classroom

- *Activity Markers:* Children's activity level correlates with their focus or distraction during play activities. When children are engaged, materials and activities hold their attention. If children are frequently moving about the room or conflict is regularly occurring in specific areas in your classroom, it is likely children are not focusing on their activities, so it is time to redesign the space.
- *Noise Level Markers:* Noise levels indicate children's level of engagement in the classroom. A low hum indicates a healthy classroom in which children are focused on their play. Silent or very noisy classrooms indicate that you should look around and see what the children are doing.
- *Movement Markers:* In calm classrooms, children use walking feet to move between spaces. Running, throwing, and other quick movements occur infrequently. When caregivers address children's movements, they walk over to the child to communicate in a dyad (one caregiver, one child) using strength-based language to problem solve together.

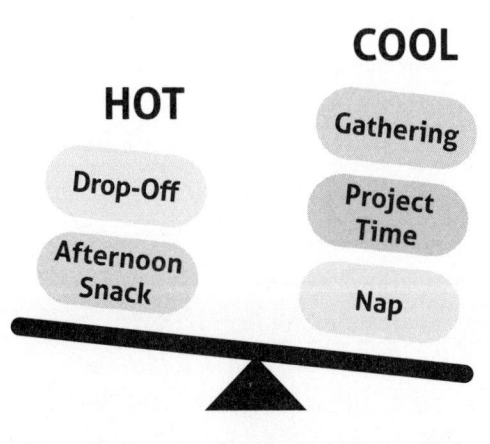

Figure 6.1. Example of Hot and Cool Times of Day

PILLAR TWO: ATTACHMENT AND CAREGIVING RELATIONSHIPS

Classroom Values that Influence Classroom Markers

- *Risk:* It is important that classrooms and outdoor spaces allow children to challenge themselves. When caregivers restrict all risk in the program, children become frustrated, then act out. Monitor and allow for spaces where children can challenge their physical and cognitive development. Both too much or too little challenge can cause frustration. When children are becoming frustrated, it is often a sign that they are not ready for the activity. Support and encourage children to continue to try, but do not complete the activity for them. Regarding physical activities, do not place children where they cannot get themselves out or down.
- *Safety:* Ensure that materials and toys are clean and include all parts. Dirty and broken materials and toys send messages about the emotional health of the classroom. Children and adults see and internalize messages about value, belonging, and self-worth from their environments.
- *Classroom Community:* Caregivers ensure that children are respectful and kind to each other. They use strength-based language and short, individual conversations to help children build a respectful community.

TABLE 6.1. TAKING THE CLASSROOM TEMPERATURE

TIME	ACTIVITY	TEMPERATURE	FEELING
8:00 am	Morning Drop-Off		
8:20 am	Morning Gathering		
8:50 am	Transition to Activities		

www.redleafpress.org/scm/6-1.pdf

In addition to monitoring your classroom's temperature, learn to recognize children's emotional states and use the classroom environment to help children self-regulate. Nurturing zones allow children to work toward self-regulating their emotions. These may be physical spaces in the classroom that are soft, cozy, or quiet with few distractions where children can feel big in a small space or see less of the movement in the classroom.

Make sure these spaces are not cluttered, as clutter invites emotional dysregulations when children have no place to rest their eyes and calm their energy. Shelves should have enough materials to engage children but with space between each material to allow children to reflect on their choices. Many great books about designing spaces for young children are available; we recommend *Designs for Living and Learning* by Deb Curtis and Margie Carter (Redleaf Press 2015).

Final Thoughts

Strength-based classrooms begin with healthy relationships between and among all the individuals who spend a portion of their lives together in the classroom. Secure relationships and attachments are essential to the mental health and wellbeing of each child. Forming respectful reciprocal relationships takes both time and energy. Creating environments where all members of the community thrive begins with caregivers forming strong dyadic relationships with each child, fostered by the caregiver's own sense of wellbeing. Strength-based practices support healthy classroom climates, which include strong communication skills between and among members of the classroom community and a strong understanding of the emotional temperature of the classroom. Much like a conductor, caregivers steer the emotional energy in their classrooms through their intentional actions and reflections.

Taking Action

What Caregivers Can Do

- Provide responsive, nurturing care to each child in your care.
- Leave your personal problems at the door and make yourself emotionally available to the children in your care.
- Introduce emotion words through songs, books, and everyday discussions.
- Take observational notes if you are concerned about a child's social and emotional development.

Reflection and Application

- Reflect on how you can lovingly connect each day with the children in your care.

- During what time of day do you notice a change in the temperature of the classroom?
- What strength-based practices can you use to assist a child who is having trouble self-regulating?

CHAPTER 7

Pillar Three: Understanding Concerning Behaviors

The more healthy relationships a child has, the more likely he will be to recover from trauma and thrive. Relationships are the agents of change and the most powerful therapy is human love.
—*Bruce D. Perry,* The Boy Who Was Raised as a Dog: And Other Stories from a Child Psychiatrist's Notebook

Children enter our care with varying degrees of mental health and wellbeing. No matter their degree of wellness, all children have the right to a loving, safe, and secure childhood. Unfortunately, we know that many children come to us exhibiting symptoms of developmental disorders or having experienced trauma. So how do we as responsive caregivers help children adjust behaviors that impede their relationships with adults and peers, increase their ability to participate in everyday classroom activities, and improve their capacity to learn and develop new developmental skills? Out of concern for the children, many care providers ask how they might recognize when children need referrals for diagnostic assessment. This is one of many questions that makes understanding mental health and wellbeing important for early care providers.

State-licensed professionals follow a complex process in determining a diagnosis, and they are trained in using diagnostic tools as a guide when working in a professional capacity with children and their families. In chapter 2, we discussed the three main diagnostic manuals: DSM-5, ICD-10, and DC:0–5. As we look at the diagnostic classification of mental health and developmental disorders in infants and young children, we will refer to information gathered from the DC:0–5. This diagnostic manual is designed to help mental health professionals and other trained professionals assess the mental health and developmental needs of young children. The information shared in this book is a general overview of the mental health disorders commonly seen in infants and young children. Please note that this book is intended for educational purposes only, not for making any diagnosis or treatment plan. Classification is a lengthy and detailed process requiring trained professionals who have a clear understanding of the diagnostic process and the developmental features of each disorder. For more information on the DC:0–5, visit the Zero to Three website at www.zerotothree.org.

When the child presents symptoms and referrals are made, the health care or mental health clinician begins an ongoing process of diagnostic formulation. The clinician or mental health professional observes the child and collects information over time from multiple sources, including the caregivers at child care and at home, within the context of family and community. Cultural expectations and expressions of emotion vary greatly, so clinicians also assess the family's cultural background and its influence on the child's presenting symptoms. As clinicians begin to make their diagnosis, they use a variety of information, such as the child's presenting symptoms, current developmental state, cultural background, interpersonal relationships, how the child adapts from home to early care, the level of family functioning, and the child's degree of attachment. For example, the child may present symptoms at home but not in the child care environment. Understanding that symptoms are present in one setting but not another will help the mental health professional begin to narrow a potential diagnosis. To gain a complete understanding of the child's functioning and their relationships with others, clinicians begin an extensive process of assessing the child in a wide range of areas and in a variety of environmental settings. Part of this process includes interviewing the parents and sometimes other adults who spend large portions of the day with the child, including professional caregivers.

To make a complete and comprehensive diagnosis, the clinician assesses the child's competencies along the developmental continuum, looking for patterns in the child's abilities to adapt and function. It is not uncommon for clinicians or a clinical team to spend time in a child care setting, observing and assessing the child on a variety of indicators, including how the child interacts with adults and peers, and exhibits motor activity, sensory sensitivity, behavior, and navigation within the child care setting. An assessment may include the child's physical and mental health, temperament, and learning style, the age at which the symptoms began, and the child's relationship with their caregivers. The clinician will assess the child's exposure to ACEs, such as the death of a parent, a sudden change in their living situation, or local or community violence. If an ACE is identified, the mental health professional will assess how this event might be contributing to the child's presenting symptoms. Lastly, mental health professionals look to see if the presenting symptoms are causing distress to both the child and their family or if they interfere with the child's relationships with others, impair their interactions in everyday activities, or limit their ability to learn and develop new skills. As you can see, a clinical assessment is very extensive; therefore, any information you can provide about the child, such as their developmental progression, classroom behavior, engagement in activities, and relationships with adults and peers, will be useful to clinicians as they begin to assess a young child in your care.

Diagnostic Classification

Mental health professionals apply general classification symptoms from a professional diagnostic manual to make a formal diagnosis. Clinicians treating children ages birth to five years generally use the DC:0–5 to assist in making a diagnosis. Diagnostic manuals identify a wide range of mental health disorders classified by common features or symptoms. For example, children with anxiety disorders commonly show symptoms of agitation, worry, and distress. Classification also considers when symptoms first appeared. For example, in sensory processing disorders, a child at birth may present sensitivity to noise or have difficulty being soothed by their caregiver. Disorders such as depressive mood disorders are generally diagnosed in children after the age of three. Classification of disorders also examines the progression or regression of symptoms and the length of time symptoms have been present. It's important to note that it is not uncommon for children with mental health and developmental delays to receive more than one diagnosis.

For the purpose of this book, we briefly discuss mental health disorders commonly seen in our early care settings, including autism spectrum disorder (ASD), attention deficit hyperactivity disorder (ADHD), sensory processing disorders, anxiety disorders, and mood disorders.

Autism Spectrum Disorders

Autism spectrum disorder is classified in the DC:0–5 under neurodevelopmental disorders. According to the Autism and Developmental Disabilities Monitoring Network Report funded by the CDC, in 2020 approximately one in fifty-four eight-year-olds in the United States were diagnosed with autism (CDC 2020a). This in an increase in numbers from previous national projections. The CDC reports that boys are four times more likely to be diagnosed with ASD than girls. It also reports that one-third of the children with ASD who had IQ scores available were also diagnosed with an intellectual disability. Autism affects all socioeconomic and ethnic groups, and the increase in the prevalence of the diagnosis is primarily due to earlier identification. According to the DC:0–5, children are not typically diagnosed until they are at least eighteen months of age (Zero to Three 2016). These are some of the ASD symptoms young children may present:

- limited or atypical social and emotional interactions
- reduced or limited attention to shared activities
- reduced or limited verbal and nonverbal skills
- reduced or limited following or understanding of gestures
- eye contact may appear atypical, or the child turns away from others in social situations
- repetitive motor and speech patterns
- rigid fixation on routines and resistance to change

Early and accurate diagnosis of ASD is essential so interventions can begin as soon as possible. If you have any concerns about a child regressing to a previous developmental stage or observe signs of repetitive or limited behaviors, be sure to discuss your concerns with the child's parent. If you observe signs of ASD, remember that young children are still developing social-emotional and communications skills, and this can make an accurate early diagnosis difficult. When observing children in your classroom, consider too that many of these behaviors are symptomatic of other mental health disorders, including ADHD.

Attention Deficit Hyperactivity Disorder

Early child care settings are noisy and busy, full of energetic and curious children. When looking at the presenting symptoms of ADHD, clinicians differentiate between typical and atypical behavior. In children with ADHD, atypical behaviors such as overactivity, impulsivity, and inattention will be more pervasive, persistent, and extreme than in typical children, and the child will present symptomatic behaviors in more than one setting, such as at child care and at home. These are some symptoms of ADHD:

- inattentive to details in play and classroom activities
- demonstrates difficulty following directions and verbal requests from adults
- avoids activities that require attention and prolonged focus
- often distracted by sounds or other interactive activities
- often forgets things
- frequently squirms and fidgets and has difficulty sitting for long periods of time
- makes excessive noise

Children who present symptoms of ADHD are often at risk for school expulsion. Current research tells us how harmful it is for children to be expelled, which makes early intervention, prevention, and strength-based classroom management critical for children's mental health and wellbeing. Children with this diagnosis exhibit limited participation in everyday, developmentally expected activities. This disorder can impair the child's ability to learn and develop new skills and interfere with their development. In addition, the family's relationships with others can be strained.

Sensory Processing Disorder

This disorder is identified in infants and young children who present persistent and pervasive symptoms of over-response or under-response when regulating sensory input. Sensitivities result in significant distress for the child or impairment of the child and their family; the child's relationships and everyday activities may be limited by this disorder, along with their participation in developmentally expected activities or routines. Sensory sensitivity can present in different sensory domains, including visual, auditory, tactile, olfactory, taste, or vestibular sensation (movement through space). Symptoms of this disorder can also present in more than one environment, such as home, early care, or community settings. In an early learning setting, children may exhibit an intense or exaggerated response to stimuli or show a minimal or limited response to normal age-related stimuli, such as sudden or unusual noises. Because child care settings are inherently busy and noisy places, children with this disorder can become easily overwhelmed. As a caregiver, your partnership with the child's family is critical as you work together to provide nurturing and responsive care. Careful observation and modification of your learning environment is essential to the wellbeing of children with sensory processing disorders. Chapter 11 includes a variety of strength-based strategies to modify your classroom. These strength-based approaches and activities will help you meet the needs of all the young children in your care.

Anxiety Disorders

Many infants and young children experience brief episodes of anxiety but quickly recover. Adults often believe that children will outgrow their fears and anxiety, which is true in many cases, but for children with persistent and pervasive symptoms of fear and anxiety, this belief can be a barrier that keeps the child from receiving age-appropriate support. Typically, children around seven or eight months begin to show symptoms of separation anxiety. For example, they might cry and reach out to their primary caregiver when dropped off at child care or cry and look away in the presence of an unfamiliar adult. As they become more familiar with the child care staff or a new adult, their symptoms quickly diminish. Children who demonstrate fear of an unfamiliar adult and separation anxiety show a strong attachment to their primary caregiver. Such anxious responses are developmentally appropriate for infants and young children and are distinct from symptoms of more persistent and pervasive anxiety disorders.

Assessing and diagnosing distressing anxiety in infants and young children is challenging because very young children are unable to verbalize their internal experiences. Left unaddressed, children with feelings of worry, fear, and anxiety feel alone, and their brains remain in a state of distress. These situations often leave adults feeling powerless to comfort the child or relieve them of their anxious and distressful feelings. As children begin to verbalize or act out their fears and worry through play, clinicians become more equipped to form a diagnosis and treatment plan. Anxiety symptoms in young children may include becoming easily agitated, irritable, or restless, and having difficulty falling and staying asleep. When assessing for a diagnosis of an anxiety disorder, the clinician also needs to look at the temperament and disposition of the child, as the characteristics of temperament may indicate that a child is more at risk for anxiety disorders. Risk factors, such as long periods of toxic stress due to physical, emotional, or sexual abuse and homelessness, also increase the child's vulnerability to feelings of fear and anxiety. Symptoms of anxiety are often seen in children with mood disorders, adding to the difficulty in diagnosing these two mental health disorders.

Mood Disorders

The symptoms of mood disorders can be extreme, so therefore the safety and wellbeing of everyone in the child care environment, including caregivers, other children, and the identified child, must be considered. Similar to anxiety disorder, children present agitated, irritable, and restless emotions and have difficulty falling and staying asleep. With mood disorders, children can exhibit periods of anger, rage, aggression, feelings of worthlessness, and profound sadness. Children with mood disorders are often stigmatized and excluded from typical everyday activities. Young children with this disorder are not easily comforted by caregivers, and they exhibit limited ability to self-regulate. The intensity and pervasiveness of these anxiety and mood disorders means early treatment and prevention plans are critical to the mental health and wellbeing of the child.

Outside Effects on Mental Health

As we've mentioned throughout this book, relationships are central to children's mental health and wellbeing. We know that stable, secure, and predictable relationships and environments provide the highest quality of care for infants and young children. As we look at the interaction between child and caregiver, it is important to note that both caregiver and child contribute to the emotional quality of the relationship. When clinicians are assessing a child for mental health issues, they examine the child within the context of the caregiving relationship. Clinicians observe the interactions between the caregiver and child in both structured and unstructured naturalistic settings to gain a better understanding of the issues and note how the child adapts and presents symptoms in multiple settings.

When assessing a child, the clinician takes a close look at the effectiveness of the caregiving relationship, including the adult's attitude toward the caregiving role, their emotional availability and responsiveness to the child's needs, their tolerance to the changing responsibilities of caring for the child, and their overall functioning. Responsive caregivers understand the important role they play in providing nurturing care. They consider their sphere of influence in fostering a strength-based early learning environment.

When assessing young children, clinicians also examine the physical wellbeing and health conditions that may influence the child and their presenting symptoms. For example, long-term health issues or hospitalization may limit the child's play experiences and hence their ability to make or keep friendships. Likewise, the caregiver and child relationship is influenced by the type, duration, and acuity of the child's medical conditions and the subsequent care the child needs. Therefore, taking into consideration physical wellbeing and health conditions is important to the diagnostic process. Here are some physical and health conditions that can affect the child's mental health:

- chronic or acute medical conditions
- intermittent or long-term hospitalization
- reactions to medications, including sluggishness, itching, or digestive problems
- conditions due to preterm birth
- prenatal conditions such as congenital malformations or genetic abnormalities
- poor prenatal care, including exposure to toxins like alcohol or drugs
- exposure to a traumatizing medical procedure
- physical injury such as a broken arm or leg
- colic
- allergies, including to foods
- cancers and tumors

Likewise, the environment in which a child grows up has a large impact on their overall mental health and wellbeing. Childhood experiences can potentially either positively or negatively affect the child's ability to connect with others, engage in everyday activities, and learn and develop new skills. Because infants and young children are dependent on adults for their basic care, they are especially vulnerable to psychosocial stressors. Stressors are intense events or lasting circumstances, such as living in poverty and exposure to violence or abuse, a parent with mental illness, or neglectful care. Clinicians gather information on the child's history and exposure to ACEs, knowing that these experiences influence the overall mental health and wellbeing of the child.

Through a thorough assessment of the child's environment and history, clinicians can evaluate the child's sense of resiliency and ability to cope and manage change. Additionally, identifying the stressors in a child's life assists the mental health professional in making a diagnosis and treatment plan that promotes the child's protective factors. Caregivers play an important role in providing protective factors for the child in their care and helping to mitigate the impact of stressors. Responsive caregivers partner with parents to support and nurture the child. Additionally, caregivers can help children build resiliency skills that will better equip them to understand and cope with environmental stressors.

Final Thoughts

Because interpersonal relationships are central to a child's development and wellbeing, your role in the process is critically important. Keeping parents informed when you become concerned about the child's developmental trajectory will be helpful in early detection of disorders. *Unfortunately,* many individuals hesitate to receive help or a diagnosis for their child due to the stigma that still exists surrounding mental illness. We know that early detection for mental disorders and developmental delays makes a positive impact on the child's overall development. You can play an important part through careful documentation and assessment of the child along the developmental continuum tool used in your practice.

Once a clinician has assessed a child, they will decide if further assessment is needed and which treatments, if any, are recommended. Treatment plans often include a team of professionals as well as the child's loved ones and care providers. Many of an individual's symptoms can be dramatically reduced with the support of family and friends. Mental health professionals can also refer the family to local support groups that provide additional protective factors for the child and their family. The National Alliance on Mental Illness (NAMI) holds family support groups across the United States to provide education and hope to families with a loved one living with mental illness. To locate a family support group near you, visit NAMI at www.nami.org. Learning more about mental illness and offering age-appropriate, strength-based practices in your child care setting can foster a child's social and emotional skills and resiliency, and hopefully set the child on a trajectory to a happy, healthy life.

Taking Action

What Caregivers Can Do

- Know your agency policies for referrals to specialists.
- Keep accurate and up-to-date documentation of each child to share with parents.
- Create role-playing scenarios to practice conversations with parents.

Reflection and Application

- What strength-based approaches can I use to promote a state of calm and sense of safety in my classroom?
- What skills and knowledge do I need to provide the best care for children with mental disorders?
- How can I partner with parents whose children have been diagnosed with disorders?
- How am I utilizing the resources in my community to meet the needs of children in my care?

CHAPTER 8

Pillar Four: Risk and Resiliency

Young children experience their world as an environment of relationships, and these relationships affect virtually all aspects of their development.
—Harvard Center for the Developing Child

The factors that surround the pillar of risk and resiliency are complex and play an important role in the child's mental health and developing sense of wellbeing. Children from birth through age five are completely dependent on the care and decisions of others for protection, food, shelter, and safety, so are therefore at greater risk for exposure to stress, abuse, and trauma. According to the National Statistics on Child Abuse from the National Children's Alliance (2020), nearly 700,000 children are abused each year in the United States. In 2018 an estimated 678,000 children were victims of abuse and neglect. Additionally, the National Children's Alliance estimates that in the same year, 1,700 children died of abuse and neglect in the United States. Of the data reported, the highest number of victims were children under the age of one. This is staggering data, yet we know that many cases of abuse and neglect go unnoticed or unreported. With the prevalence of abuse in the United States, we know that many children are living in stressful, traumatic, and sometimes life-threatening situations. We know that for optimal growth and development, children need safe, stable, and nurturing care where their basic needs are met. Young children need support and care from responsive caregivers who can provide a safe learning environment in which they can grow and thrive.

As adults working with young children, we are responsible for assisting children in developing coping and resiliency skills while equipping them to manage varying degrees of adverse experiences. Therefore, gaining a deeper understanding of risk and resiliency will better equip caregivers in providing nurturing, responsive care to our youngest and more vulnerable children.

Risk Factors

According to the CDC (2020a), children younger than age four are the most at-risk population overall, with children birth through age two ranking highest in both risk factors and incidents. This is primarily due to the high needs of our youngest children, the lack of parental understanding of child development and what's developmentally appropriate, and the fact that young children are still developing the ability to verbally articulate their needs to adults. Additionally, our youngest children have less exposure to community professionals than older school-age children. Children who are premature or have disabilities are also at high risk for maltreatment due to the caregiver's increased feelings of stress, isolation, and grief, along with the additional financial and emotional burdens of caregiving. Stress and trauma can be found in any socioeconomic group, but certain identified living conditions place children at greater risk. The following situations, behaviors, and living conditions might indicate that a child is at risk of stress, abuse, or trauma:

Environmental

- The child is exposed to pornography or sexual images.
- There is substance abuse, alcoholism, or mental health issues, including depression, in the home.
- Parents are young, low-income, uneducated, or single.
- The household includes transient members, including nonbiologically related adults.
- Family dysfunction is present, including domestic violence, separation, divorce, or poor parent-child or other interpersonal relationships.
- The community faces violence, limited resources, or high poverty and unemployment.

Emotional

- Parents fail to satisfy the child's basic needs for food, shelter, clothing, emotional support, and supervision.
- The child is separated from their home and placed with unfamiliar adults or in foster or social service care.
- Parents experience social isolation.

Relational

- Parents have a history of child abuse and/or neglect.
- Parents have anger issues, poor self-awareness, and poor emotional regulation.
- Parents support or justify corporal punishment or maltreatment of children.
- The parent-child relationship is insecure.
- Parents have a limited understanding of attachment and developmental needs.
- Parents have a history of depression or experience maternal or fraternal depression.

Other

- Children were born prematurely or with a disability.
- Birth mothers received little or no prenatal care while pregnant.
- The fetus was exposed to drugs, alcohol, or other toxic substances.

Health care professionals and caregivers are often the first adults outside the home who observe signs of physical and emotional trauma in children. These individuals are often mandated reporters who are legally required to report when abuse is observed or suspected. Due to many circumstances, trauma is not always visible, and abuse does not always appear in the form of visible injuries such as bruises, cuts, or broken bones. Psychological and emotional abuse, such as isolating, rejecting, or ignoring a child, are harder to prove unless directly observed by an adult. One of the first indicators that something might be wrong that mandated reporters might observe is a dramatic change in children's behavior, such as sensitivity to touch, ongoing crying, angry outbursts, or lack of engagement in typical activities. Such changes in a child's behavior strongly indicate that something has changed in a child's life. The changes may be typical and nothing to worry about, but they may also be red flags that something else is going on in the child's world. We must carefully observe and document events. If a caregiver becomes concerned about a child's wellbeing, they must safeguard the child by taking proper steps and following agency protocol. Every state has mandated reporting requirements. These are some of the ways to prepare to report:

- taking annual, professional development training on mandated reporting
- reviewing your program's protocols for mandated reporting
- gathering contact information about the child for your call
- making sure your notes are factual regarding what you heard or saw
- knowing your mandated reporting agencies are there to help you
- waiting to ask the child to tell what happened until they are in the presence of a social services staff member
- keeping information confidential from other teachers, parents, or staff in your program, except as identified in your protocol

Reporting child abuse is an emotional experience for caregivers. After the reporting is complete, be sure to set aside time for yourself to process your feelings and your concerns for the welfare of the child and family. Attending to yourself and practicing self-care is important when child abuse reports need to be made. Making mandated reports is difficult but essential as we advocate for and protect the safety and wellbeing of the children in our care.

Adverse Experiences

In today's world, we are all affected by stress and trauma to one degree or another. The ACEs study conducted between 1995 to 1997 (see figure 8.1) identifies that abuse, neglect, and household dysfunction caused the most profound and lasting adverse impacts on developing children. The ACEs study also estimates that 62 percent of adults surveyed had experienced at least one ACE during childhood, and nearly one-quarter report having experienced three or more ACEs (CDC 2020a). Children can be exposed to more than one ACE at a time or multiple ACEs during the course of their childhood. Abuse is identified in the forms of physical, emotional, or sexual. Neglect is classed in the ACEs study as both physical and emotional. Lastly, household dysfunction includes parental incarceration, mental illness, substance abuse, violence toward a partner or family member, and parental absence due to separation or divorce (CDC 2020a).

Stress and Trauma

Often spoken of simultaneously, stress and trauma have the power to influence and shape the developing child and alter or disrupt the architecture of the developing brain. Stress and trauma are experienced differently by each child. Stress is an emotional feeling or physical tension felt in the body, whereas trauma, or traumatic events, produces either a psychological injury or physical or emotional pain. Trauma can be a single event, a series of events, or a set of reoccurring events. Stress is identified by degrees of intensity from mild to tolerable to toxic. Each degree of stress produces varying degrees of strain or tension in an individual, resulting in unique responses.

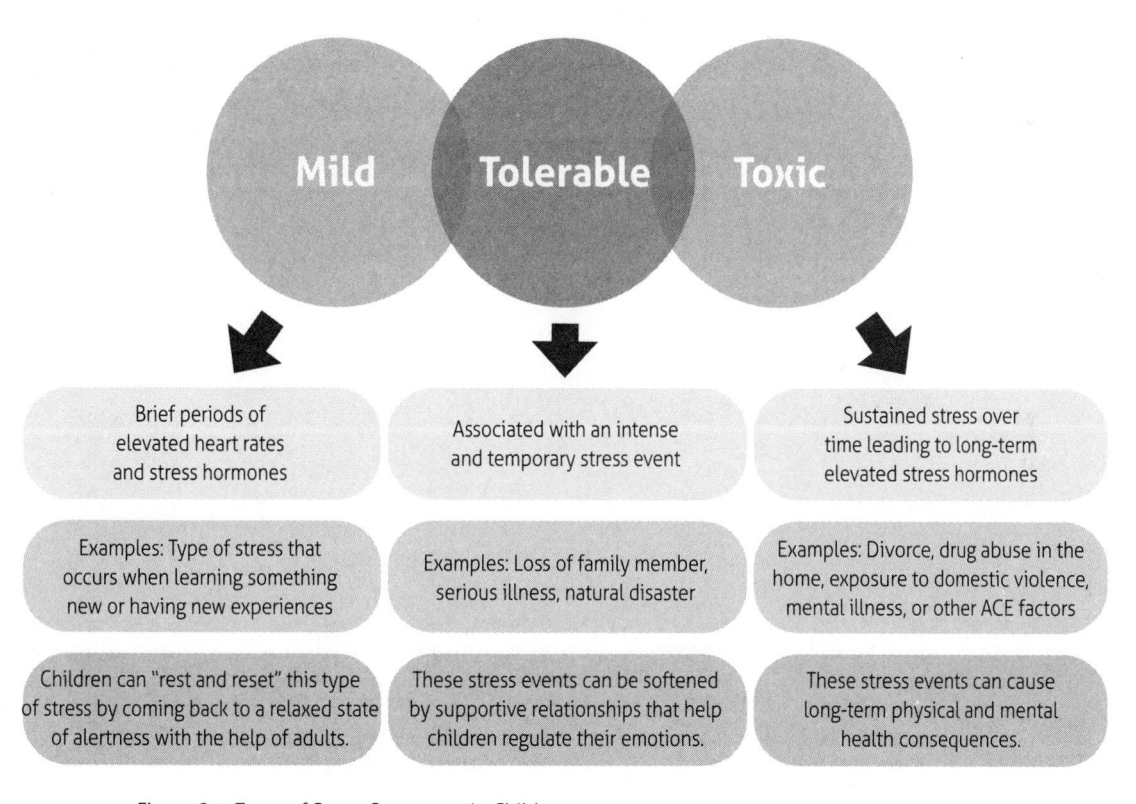

Mild — Brief periods of elevated heart rates and stress hormones
- Examples: Type of stress that occurs when learning something new or having new experiences
- Children can "rest and reset" this type of stress by coming back to a relaxed state of alertness with the help of adults.

Tolerable — Associated with an intense and temporary stress event
- Examples: Loss of family member, serious illness, natural disaster
- These stress events can be softened by supportive relationships that help children regulate their emotions.

Toxic — Sustained stress over time leading to long-term elevated stress hormones
- Examples: Divorce, drug abuse in the home, exposure to domestic violence, mental illness, or other ACE factors
- These stress events can cause long-term physical and mental health consequences.

Figure 8.1. Types of Stress Responses in Children

Mild forms of stress are temporary or brief episodes of discomfort that are quickly resolved. Typically, children adapt to mild stressors with little effort. For example, feeling uncomfortable with a wet diaper for a few minutes or saying good-bye to a parent at drop-off is often sad or upsetting for a child, but with responsive caregiving, these episodes of mild stress are quickly overcome and last only for a short period until the child is comforted and the issue is resolved.

Tolerable stress increases in intensity from mild stress and may occur for longer periods of time. Tolerable stress has the potential to activate the brain's nervous system and alert the body to move into a fight, flight, or freeze response. Examples of tolerable stress are being hospitalized, having a parent deployed in the armed services, or being in a car accident. Even though the stress is more intense than a mild stressor, the nervous system in the brain is not activated for long periods of time. The stress event itself can be intense, but the child often recovers to their prior state with the assistance of loving, stable caregivers.

Experiencing mild and tolerable stressors can help children build resiliency skills, confidence, and autonomy as they adapt to stressors and changes in their environment. Caring, nurturing environments built on a trusting relationship between child and caregiver are essential to helping the child adjust to all degrees of stress. Responsive caregivers quickly acknowledge and respond with care and compassion to the stressors children experience, helping them feel safe and loved.

Trauma can range from a onetime event, such as a loss of a loved one, to toxic stress, when an individual lives in an environment that is chronically stressful or where traumatic events repeatedly occur. Some examples of toxic stress are regularly hearing or witnessing domestic violence, enduring abuse in any form, or living in a community where violence and crime are present. Traumatic events can be caused by individual human interactions, either by a family member or through a nonfamily relationship, or from a societal, communal, or natural event or crisis, such as a flood, earthquake, or pandemic. These events can threaten the individual's life, the safety and integrity of their body, or their mental state.

The brain's nervous system is activated when exposed to situations of extreme and prolonged toxic stress and trauma, and prolonged activation of this stress response can adversely affect the developing brain. When children live with toxic stress, their brains are always on alert to fight, flee, or freeze. A child may feel overwhelmed or helpless when a traumatic event occurs, or struggle to integrate the emotional experience into their previous sense of wellbeing. Children are also more likely to experience multiple ACEs when living in situations that create toxic stress; for example, an alcoholic parent in the home can be extremely stressful for a child, and if the alcoholic parent's behavior escalates, the child is at risk for experiencing additional ACEs.

Our history and exposure to past traumatic events influences how we manage new and ongoing stressful or adverse experiences. Coping strategies, access to supportive family and community members, and mental health services can all provide protective factors to both adults and children who have been exposed to traumatic events and toxic stress.

Children's responses to stress and trauma are as unique as each child and each event. For example, two siblings might respond differently to the same situation, such as domestic violence. One child might sit and cry in the corner or completely shut down, while the other tries to comfort, reassure, or even rescue the injured parent. The child's response differs by the age of the child, prior exposure to traumatic events, and their ability to interpret the event or seek safety or help. From this you can see that the youngest children, birth through age five, are more at risk. Babies, toddlers, and children with severe disabilities are extremely at risk because they are so dependent on adults for safety and survival.

The circumstances surrounding the event and how the adults around them respond to help and support the child are critical in how the event is remembered and stored in the child's brain. With neural pathways in the brain still developing, children are not able to articulate or understand their reactions to trauma, but they internalize the experiences. As adults, they may recall childhood incidents of trauma, thinking, *Why did this happen to me? What did I do to cause this? Who were the adults around me that helped me feel safe?* Often young children feel that a traumatic event is their fault and subsequently internalize feelings of shame and doubt.

Regardless of the age of the individual, prolonged periods of stress and trauma have a cumulative effect and can result in a decline in one's overall physical and mental health, leaving an individual more prone to infectious and immune-related diseases. Although children are resilient and adults may not notice their degree of stress, we know that the effect of stress on the developing brain and body is present and lasting. Its long-term effects can be referred to as an *imprint* or *thumbprint* on the body. Like an actual thumbprint, each adverse traumatic experience is unique with its own surrounding circumstances.

The Brain's Response to Trauma

Weighing just over three pounds, the human brain is a complex and amazing organ that regulates a wide range of activities: thinking, problem solving, expressing emotion, learning new tasks, mastering tasks such as walking and running, learning language, and communicating with others. The brain also organizes our thinking, stores memories and experiences, and regulates our breathing and heart rate. Ninety percent of the brain will be developed before a child enters kindergarten, which is why it is so important to understanding how both positive and negative experiences influence the developing brain. Dr. Bruce Perry (2020) states that all experiences change and influence the brain, but not all experiences are equal. Experiences such as an adult reading or playing with a child stimulates positive neural connections, while negative experiences like being hit by an adult or hearing or witnessing domestic violence strengthens negative brain connections or pathways.

Historically, little emphasis was placed on how stress and trauma affected young children, especially babies and children under the age of three. It was thought that they were too young to notice or be affected by hearing, witnessing, or being the direct victim of toxic stress and abuse. There was a feeling that they would "just get over it." But today's brain research tells us something quite the opposite: we now know that the brain's response to stress, trauma, and threats can leave a lasting imprint on the developing child. Because young children's brains during their first five years are organizing so quickly and neural pathways are being so rapidly created, exposure to stress and trauma greatly affects the architecture of the developing brain. Adverse experiences can have lasting effects on the brain's size, structure, and ability to organize, regulate emotions, focus attention, and learn.

The human brain begins to develop just four weeks after conception, making it highly sensitive to the mother's health and lifestyle factors. Maternal and environmental stress, along with exposure to neurotoxins like drugs and alcohol, can negatively affect the unborn child. Good prenatal care and healthy choices are important for the baby's optimal brain development. From birth on, the brain continues to need good nutrition as well as safe, secure, and loving living conditions.

We are born with billions of neurons that shape the brain for a lifetime. During the first three years of life, the child's brain is rapidly changing and is more flexible than during any other period. This period of brain development is called neuroplasticity, when the brain forms and reorganizes synaptic connections in response to new information, sensory stimulation, and the absence or presence of stimuli, stress, and trauma. The young brain is naturally susceptible to the pruning and stimulation called plasticity, which allows the brain to change and adapt to stimuli. The brain loves novelty and is profoundly influenced by exposure to repeated and new stimuli. Children's brains become more sophisticated as more and more connections are built. Exposure to developmentally appropriate, hands-on activities, as well as warm, loving, and responsive caregivers, strengthens the brain's pathways. We know too that windows of opportunity are present during the first five years of life when children develop key skills that last throughout their lifetime, such as recognizing sounds and learning language.

The brain is one of the most complex organs in the body and grows from the bottom up, starting with the brain stem. It is divided into three main areas: brain stem, limbic system, and the neocortex or frontal cortex. The brain stem controls heart rate, breathing, swallowing, eating, and sleeping habits. The limbic system regulates emotions, attachments, and our body's ability to feel warmth, comfort, and pain. The amygdala, which lies in the limbic system, helps us feel and perceive emotions and process memories, fears, and threats. The frontal cortex controls important analytical and complex thinking, problem solving and reasoning skills, and regulatory abilities (such as impulse control, social interaction, and self-regulation, to name a few). It helps us with emotional expression, language, memory, and judgment. Our executive function is located in the frontal cortex, which affects our ability to be flexible in our thinking, access past memories to solve problems, and manage daily life.

During periods of toxic stress and trauma, our limbic system activates the stress hormones adrenaline and cortisol. When a person senses a threat in any form, the amygdala, sometimes called the "smoke detector" of the body, instantly reacts by sending a response in the form of adrenalin throughout the brain. This adrenalin rush causes an increase in heart rate and respiration, and sends energy to our muscles, which triggers a fight, flight, or freeze response. Our brain then releases cortisol, the primary stress hormone, triggering the body to shake, tremble, go numb, or freeze. Cortisol is neither good nor bad, but surges in cortisol (during times of stress) affect our higher-order thinking.

The frontal cortex is inhibited by cortisol, so during times of stress, the brain's ability to focus, follow directions, organize thoughts, problem solve, and regulate emotions becomes temporality compromised. Therefore, an individual whose brain is in a stress response may have trouble explaining what happened, logically responding to questions, or regulating their emotions. Once the threat subsides, the brain slowly returns to its prior state, and the event is processed and stored in the amygdala as feeling, sensory, muscle, and automatic memories.

Exposure to adverse experiences can cause neural pathways to respond more quickly to any degree of threat or stress in the future. This may cause young children to have their stress response easily triggered or reactivated. This activation can compromise their brain development, as excessive activation of the stress response system takes both a mental and physical toll on the body.

Children's Response to Trauma

Unsurprisingly, children who live in stressful environments or were exposed to traumatic events have trouble adjusting to classroom environments. Children coming into our care who have experienced either a onetime traumatic event or the cumulative effects of trauma and stress demonstrate a variety of concerning behaviors and are at risk for behavioral and relationship problems, academic struggles, making emotionally unhealthy decisions, and suffering a lifetime of mental health issues. In addition, studies show that children's exposure to violence may lead to their becoming a victim of violence later in life or perpetuating violence (Office of Juvenile Justice and Delinquency Prevention 2000). A child's sensory system is also greatly affected by trauma. Their ability to hear, see, touch, and sometimes taste and smell can be decreased by witnessing or being directly exposed to stress and trauma. A child's ability to recognize cause and effect and sense or anticipate danger can be damaged by loud noises, strong visual stimuli, violent images, or other stimuli experienced during a traumatic event (NCTSN 2020).

The younger the child, the more vulnerable their developing brains are to the effects of trauma. Trauma impacts the whole child: their physical body, developing brain, emotions, and behavior. Their concerning behaviors can also range anywhere from mild to moderate to extreme. Symptoms you witness may be indicators of more serious stressors or concerns that are placing the child's development at risk. When examining the symptoms of young children in our care, it is important to look at the whole child while considering the Six Pillars. We know that like adults, children's energy levels and emotions can fluctuate by the day, but these symptoms and moods are not consistent or long-lasting. It is important when looking at the symptoms that we don't pathologize or jump to the conclusion that a child is a victim of trauma, as this is the job of medical and mental health professionals. Our job as responsive caregivers is to provide a safe, nurturing learning environment where children can grow and thrive. If indeed symptoms appear, last over time, and do not seem to improve, you may want to discuss your concerns with the proper staff members at your child care center or make referrals for a professional assessment. We spoke in detail in earlier chapters about mental health and the criteria for diagnosing developmental disorders. As we shared before, mental health diagnosing must be done by a professional mental health practitioner or specialist (see table 2.1, Professional Mental Health Practitioners and Specialists), but when early care providers witness concerning symptoms they have clearly documented over time, it is their job to make referrals to appropriate professionals. The following are behaviors that may indicate trauma in young children.

Symptoms in Children Ages Birth through Two Years:

- cries inconsolably
- does not coo or make sounds
- does not follow you with their eyes
- is not interested in playing interactive games or with toys
- spends a lot of time rocking or comforting themselves
- avoids eye contact
- does not smile; has a dull look or blank facial expression
- does not reach out to be picked up
- awakens screaming; cannot relax to fall asleep or falls asleep suddenly in the midst of noise and commotion; has trouble focusing when awake
- rejects your efforts to calm, soothe, and connect

- has poor muscle tone; flails arms and legs loosely or cannot pull up against gravity; trembles
- startles at noise, light, or touch and cannot recover
- yawns, drools, or hiccups; feels chilled or clammy; has pale or blotchy skin
- does not seem to notice or care when you leave them alone

Symptoms in Children Ages Three through Five Years:

- high sensitivity to caregiver guidance; easily upset or frequently cries
- hypervigilance
- hyperactivity
- behavioral changes such as poor self-regulation and impulsivity
- angry outbursts
- difficulty being soothed or calmed by primary caregiver
- depressive symptoms such as withdrawal or not engaging in typical classroom activities
- ambivalent to primary caregiver or parent at drop-off or pickup
- difficulty forming relationships and interacting with peers
- anxiety
- problems with sleeping, toileting, or eating
- nightmares
- physical complaints such as stomachaches, pains in body
- inappropriate touching of self and others
- difficulty focusing on learning tasks and following simple directions

Adults manage stress differently than young children. Because adults generally have more life experiences, problem-solving abilities, and communication skills, they have more sophisticated ways of coping, communicating, resolving conflict, and articulating their needs. For both adolescents and adults, stressors can trigger emotions of frustration, anger, anxiety, or nervousness, along with physical tension, which makes them feel listless, tired, restless, or unable to relax. Adolescents and adults may become more withdrawn from social interactions, avoid stressful situations, have trouble in school or work settings, or experience poor memory and concentration. Adolescents and adults may numb their feelings through drugs, alcohol, risk-taking behavior, or other negative, unhealthy, or addictive behaviors. For both children and adults, friendships and close relationships may be harmed or even severed. For any age, our ability to adapt and manage stress depends on the types, demands, severity, and duration of the stressful or traumatic events.

Resiliency and Protective Factors

The long-term effects of adverse experiences can gravely influence a young child, but when children develop resiliency skills and are surrounded by protective factors, they are better equipped to cope, adapt, and overcome stress and trauma. Protective factors include a variety of ideas, concepts, and practices with the intent of providing a safety net for children. Protective factors include responsive parents who have a developmentally appropriate understanding of child development, stable housing, positive social interactions, and a consistent medical home. Along with resiliency skills, protective factors have the potential to lessen the impact of adverse experiences by providing a safety net that helps protect the child's sense of safety, security, and wellbeing. This safety net becomes larger when more protective factors are in it. As a responsive caregiver, we must reflect on ways to enhance or enlarge all children's safety nets and protective factors, including those at high risk for stress and trauma.

The adults who provide primary care for young children, including parents and early caregivers, have the greatest impact on children's wellbeing and their development of resiliency skills. We know that resilient children develop in emotionally and physically safe home and child care environments where they receive the care and nurturing they need to grow, develop, and thrive. Building resiliency skills in young children takes time. As children's brains develop, their language and communication skills improve as they become more aware of themselves and others, which builds their empathy and caring for others and their capacity to identify and regulate their emotions. Taking care of our own emotional needs is essential as we attend to the needs of the children in our care. If your resiliency is low or you are more reactive or sensitive to the demanding needs of the child care setting, take steps to care for yourself and your needs. The more resilient you are yourself, the better you will be able to help children develop their own resiliency skills.

As a caregiver, you can model resiliency skills in the learning environment through your everyday interactions with children, centered around a strength-based philosophy. Children develop resiliency skills when early learning environments focus on the strengths and capabilities of the developing children. In a strength-based approach, problems—not the child—are seen as the problem. This philosophy believes that people can grow and change through adversity and that children can make warm, caring, loving connections that will strengthen their resiliency. Using strength-based approaches helps young children begin to internalize and believe in their ability to adapt and cope. A strength-based early learning environment places the focus on how responsive caregivers can support the child in learning to draw from their own strengths, motivation, and desire to positively resolve issues.

In a strength-based early learning environment, caregivers must approach their work with young children through the lens of the whole child. Taking the time to clearly understand the whole child and document your thoughts and observations will assist you in fostering resiliency skills. Asking yourself reflective questions, such as *What are the child's strengths? How does the child demonstrate curiosity? How does the child show concern for others?* and *How does the child express their need for human connection?* will help you gain a better understanding of the child and how they approach stress and trauma.

Often a wall of silence or secrecy surrounds families who experience mental health issues, substance abuse, violence, or dysfunction. When children are isolated from outside protective factors and their resiliency skills are limited, they are more at risk. Protective factors provide opportunities for families to break through their walls of silence and secrecy to move from a closed family system to a more open system, allowing members to receive the help they need and protect children from further trauma and abuse. We discuss open and closed family systems in chapter 9.

If the child's stress and trauma originates in their home environment, it is essential that they have access to responsive adults outside the home to support them physically and emotionally, such as caregivers, medical professionals, social service agency staff, home visitors, extended family, and friends. Because caregivers often see children daily, they provide a vital safety net. It is essential that responsive caregivers take warning signs of abuse and neglect seriously and follow their agency's proper protocols for intervening on behalf of the child.

Primary caregivers, including parents and child care providers, provide children with critical relationships that help strengthen their resiliency and protective factors. In 1990 the Search Institute began to closely examine the behaviors, relationships, and skills adolescents needed to develop and succeed in school and in life. It believes that relationships are powerful in helping children and youth develop and grow as individuals. The Search Institute referred to these connections as developmental relationships. It found that developmental relationships positively influence youth by helping them make a positive impact on the world, learn more about themselves, and foster deeper connections to the important people in their lives (Search Institute 2020). The Search Institute's work identified forty developmental assets for adolescents and has now expanded the developmental assets to school-age children and children ages three to five. To learn more about the Search Institute and their forty developmental assets, visit their website at www.search-institute.org. The Search Institute found that those children and youth displaying many of these forty developmental assets demonstrate many positive attributes: they do better in school, have healthier boundaries, promote community values, show leadership, have positive relationships with family and peers, and are less likely to participate in risk-taking behaviors. Building and strengthening children's internal and external assets, including their primary relationships, helps increase protective factors for all youth and children.

As we reiterate throughout this book, we believe that relationships are central to a child's learning, mental health, and wellbeing. As we begin to identify specific protective factors caregivers can incorporate into their practice, we must always consider the whole child by first examining their current state of wellbeing, then building on their strengths through teaching, modeling, and caring for them. The following conditions allow children to develop strength-based protective factors both at home and in child care settings:

- Children are supported physically, mentally, socially, and emotionally by family members, caregivers, and other nurturing adults.
- Families have healthy boundaries with children and appropriate expectations of them.
- Children are given opportunities to play and be creative.

- Children are given opportunities to explore their curiosity and interests at home and in child care settings.
- Children are given opportunities to develop and master new skills.
- Children are taught social and emotional skills through literature and interactions with others, including caring adults.
- Children are heard and respected by caring adults.
- Children participate in age-appropriate religious activities or practices that nurture spiritual development.
- Children participate in family activities at home.
- Adults quickly respond to the needs of children in a calm and reassuring manner.
- Children explore ways to express and regulate their emotions and build close relationships with adults and peers.
- Adults use strength-based language with children when resolving conflict.
- Adults model strength-based decision-making.
- Adults read books to children that show children overcoming obstacles, demonstrating care and compassion for others, and working together to solve problems and build friendships.
- Caregivers set age-appropriate classroom expectations.

Final Thoughts

In responsive caregiving settings, we provide opportunities for children to learn how to adapt, manage their emotions, and build resiliency skills. We know that living in a toxic home environment and being exposed to trauma takes a large toll on developing children and their brains. For some children, child care and school are their only safe havens from the stress and trauma of their home or community. Each child has the right to feel safe and secure with their basic needs for food, shelter, and love provided. Therefore, our role as caregivers is to respond to the needs of children in a loving, caring, and stable manner to help them develop the resiliency skills and protective factors they need to safely navigate life's stressors.

Unfortunately, we know that many children experience stress and trauma. The more caregivers can do to provide protective factors and strength-based practices in their early care setting, the more children will develop resiliency skills. Helping children feel safe and secure in your care is essential. The more you can do to help children feel that they are safe, secure, and loved, the better it is for *all* children. It is essential that responsive caregivers take the warning signs of abuse and neglect seriously and follow the proper protocols of their agency for intervening on behalf of children. When you know a child is at risk, seek appropriate professionals to support yourself, the child, and their family. Working together, you can provide an optimal safety net for all involved.

Taking Action

What Caregivers Can Do

- Consider ways to introduce social and emotional language into your practice.
- Plan everyday activities that encourage children to build relationships with you as well as with peers.
- Review your agency's policy for making referrals if abuse or neglect is suspected.
- Create a list of social and protective services in case a referral is needed.
- Take annual mandated reporting classes.

Reflection and Application

- What emotions surface for you when stress and trauma are discussed?
- How do your feelings of protection for the child affect your emotional availability to stay present in your caregiving role?
- How do you promote protective factors and resiliency in the children in your care?

CHAPTER 9

Pillar Five: Family Relationships and Culture

Each child's family has its own composition and history, its own strengths and its own ways of coping with stress and adversity.
—The Center on the Social and Emotional Foundations for Early Learning

Healthy relationships, family, and culture are at the center of child wellbeing. We believe that responsive caregiving means supporting families with a strength-based approach. Strength-based approaches view families as bringing their own unique skills and understandings into early childhood programs. As caregivers, we acknowledge these strengths by recognizing that every family has culture, and every culture comes with its own values and knowledge that support families in navigating their world.

Also used in social work, the strength-based approach is designed to reframe how we approach children and families. Many historical and current models come from a deficit approach that identifies what is needed rather than what is already present. Deficit models focus on what is wrong with a child or family and how they need to change their actions or behaviors. These models are so ingrained in our educational, medical, and social systems that we fail to recognize how they view and approach families. For example, in early education, the deficit model speaks about what a child needs to learn, what they do not know or cannot yet do. A strength-based model approaches learning through the lens of what a child already knows, and reflects on how to offer experiences that build on existing knowledge. While the differences may seem small, what a child needs to learn versus how a child builds on their prior knowledge greatly changes our approach to learning and caring for children. The consistent use of the deficit model significantly influences the way society currently sees children, culture, and race. These models systematically disprivilege groups of children and families, diminishing their access to opportunities.

Framing Cultural Strengths

Every child is born into a family, community, and societal culture. A family's experiences within different cultural circles influences the trajectory of a child's development. Social-cultural approaches to development acknowledge that development is both environmental and biological. Lev Vygotsky was a pioneer of the social-cultural approach, showing that all children's development occurs within the social and cultural environment of a specific time in history. Contemporary researchers further acknowledge that all experiences occur within a social context and that both societal messages and environmental structures influence development. The larger the structural challenges are, such as systemic racism, the greater the effect on family resources and wealth and, likewise, relationships between caregivers and young children.

We must employ a cultural lens if we are to respect and work with families using a strength-based approach. Particular attention is focused on a child's individual experiences, the family's unique circumstances, and how culture and history have shaped them. Many aspects of mental health and wellbeing are connected not just to an individual's personal lived experiences but the experiences of a community and culture over time. Ensuring that our programs are culturally safe spaces is important in our work with families, which we do by paying attention to power relationships at individual, familial, communal, and societal levels. When families walk through the doors of our programs, we want to acknowledge that they bring more than themselves—they also bring their family and community experiences and histories.

Understanding Family Views about Mental Health and Family System Theory

Caregivers start their work by acknowledging that every family has unique strengths and funds of knowledge that caregivers can build on to support young children's health and wellbeing. Strength-based approaches move the focus away from the deficit model of viewing a child who displays complex behaviors as lacking something. The strength-based approach asks, *What is working for this child/family? How can I build on a family's strengths? How can I help add to this family's skill and protective factors?*, rather than asking, *What does this child/family need to learn or do better?* By using the strength-based approach, we develop new patterns of thought in which we see family as partners who are teaching us how to engage with them. This changes the dynamics in classrooms and programs.

This is what our work then becomes:

- creating relationships between and alongside families that support the building of classroom and program community to foster each child's development, the wellbeing of the family within the community, and positive parent-child interactions
- inviting families into culturally respectful dialogues that include their participation in decisions about their experiences in programs and with the program's practices and policies
- engaging each family's unique skills as part of their contribution to the children, the classroom, the program, and the community
- understanding that each family has a unique view of mental health and that their models of it, ways of expressing comfort, and ideas about child development may be very different than our own, and that this is part of the family's strength

Family views on mental health vary greatly. The concepts of mental health or illness still carry a societal stigma shaped by a lack of understanding of the factors contributing to these conditions. Mental illness is still viewed by some families as secretive and shameful. These beliefs arise from models in which mental health and illness are seen as character or personality issues rather than biological symptoms requiring medical treatment. The belief that mental health is not connected to biological health is still widespread, and admission of a mental health diagnosis or condition can lead families to feel stigmatized in some communities. Different culture and communities have different approaches to understanding mental health. As caregivers, we must keep in mind that families view and react to mental health issues in more than one way, which is why engaging in strength-based approaches in our early care and education community is so important.

As we work with families, we also must consider each family's internal dynamics. The family system theory helps us increase our understanding of how families function and why some families are open to supports and others are more self-contained or closed. Open and closed family systems are defined by the willingness of each individual family member to adapt and react to change. It is important to recognize that open and closed family systems exist across all cultures and economic levels. In a closed family system, members oppose change and strictly maintain the status quo. Changes in the form of new ideas, family roles, experiences, or ways of thinking are met with resistance. Think about being in a room where the windows and doors are covered and shut. When changes occur, there is no adaptation. Routines and rules do not bend or adjust within the family. Communication is difficult because ideas remain fixed. In closed family systems, secrets flourish. Closed family systems remain isolated and often experience shame.

An open family system supports and embraces change and personal growth. New ideas, experiences, friendships, and community involvement are welcomed. While changes or decisions may be difficult, families adapt due to the openness of their family system. The unique skills and talents of each family member are valued, respected, and celebrated. In open family systems, routines and rules adapt over time as the family evolves as a system. Here are additional characteristics of open and closed family systems:

Open Family Systems

- Family members are valued and individual differences are respected.
- Family members have close, loving relationships with each other.
- Conflict is resolved in mutually beneficial ways.
- Family members contribute to decisions, and everyone has a voice in the process.

- Individuals share ideas and openly communicate their needs.
- Rules, routines, and family roles are consistent and intentional.
- Members of the family play to their strengths.
- Families have meaningful connections and relationships outside the home that change and evolve over time.
- Thinking in families changes over time, influenced by the dynamic of the family and the context of the time, place, and space in which they move.

Closed Family Systems

- Individuals have limited personal freedom.
- A single individual is responsible for decision making.
- Decisions involving all members of the family are not discussed as a group.
- There is little communication among family members.
- Rules and routines can be rigid, inconsistent, or arbitrary.
- Family members do not create connections or relationships beyond the family system.
- Differing opinions are not tolerated and can cause a family member to be cut off from the family system.
- There is a right way of thinking, acting, or behaving.

Although change is difficult for most people, the type of family system, either open or closed, significantly influences how a family functions and responds to change. For example, if a family is faced with devastating news about the mental health of a child, an open family system is more apt to work together with caregivers and support services by asking questions and advocating for their child. In a closed family system, more often than not, devastating news is met with resistance or hesitation in contacting specialized support services.

Your relationship with the families in your care is critical, especially during difficult and challenging periods. Caregivers who have built strong relationships with families of either system play a pivotal role in how families respond in challenging situations. We want to prevent families from denying their children the services they need to grow and thrive. Through understanding the dynamics of family systems, we are better equipped to respond to their needs, which strengthens their protective factors.

Supporting Families through a Cultural Lens

In implementing strength-based approaches to mental health and well-being in children, we must first look at families through the lens of culture, understanding that culture is a part of child development. Barbara Rogoff, author of *The Cultural Nature of Human Development*, reminds us that we must move beyond our own assumptions about culture when working with families and reflecting on views of development. There are four key actions we can take:

- Move beyond ethnocentrisms to consider different perspectives.
- Consider diverse cultural goals for the child's development.
- Recognize the value of the knowledge of both insiders and outsiders of a specific cultural community.
- Systemically and open-mindedly revisit our inevitably local understandings so they become more encompassing (Rogoff 2003).

Our most successful conversations with families occur when we establish respectful reciprocal relationships with them that can build over time and focus on strength-based approaches to engagement. When communicating with parents, caregivers frame conversations in terms of what they notice are children's strengths. Parents need to hear about their children's successes to build trusting relationships with caregivers.

TABLE 9.1. STRENGTH-BASED VERSUS DEFICIT-BASED APPROACHES WHEN ENGAGING CHILDREN

STRENGTH-BASED APPROACHES WHEN ENGAGING CHILDREN	DEFICIT-BASED APPROACHES WHEN ENGAGING CHILDREN
Empowering children to make choices	Controlling how choices are made
Engaging by asking open-ended questions and waiting for responses	Asking yes-or-no questions or expecting a right or correct answer
Encouraging peer-to-peer interactions	Intervening in peer-to-peer interactions by directing what needs to happen next
Offering process-focused activities that provide opportunities to make, experiment, and discover without a fixed outcome in mind	Giving directions for behavior and choosing activities that have a product, objective, or behavior in mind rather than a process

Encouraging curiosity and exploration	Strongly mandating that children follow directions
Incorporating children's interests into the classroom's daily life	Designing or offering the main curriculum without the children's input
Presenting hands-on activities and experiences	Presenting curriculum with pre-determined outcomes
Focusing on and acknowledging what a child can do	Focusing on what a child cannot do or does not know

When we as caregivers have concerns about children, we make sure to respectfully address them by choosing appropriate times and places to have conversations. A respectful way to ask a parent or a family for a time together could be, "When could we spend some time together so I can learn more about Thomas and ways to further support his engagement in classroom?" Some caregivers wonder whether using a strength-based perspective means never having complex conversations about how children are navigating classroom experiences. Strength-based perspectives encourage honest conversations about children's actions and behaviors that build on children's strengths. Sometimes complex conversations are difficult, and parents may become defensive or unwilling to hear our observations about their children's behavior. Finding the right time to present our observations or concerns takes practice as well as sensitivity to the individual and cultural needs of the family. These conversations become easier when we have built respectful reciprocal relationships with parents.

TABLE 9.2. STRENGTH-BASED VERSUS DEFICIT-BASED APPROACHES

STRENGTH-BASED APPROACHES	DEFICIT-BASED APPROACHES
First considering the child's skills, personality, and strengths when thinking of them	First considering the child's issues, behaviors, or problems when thinking of them
Building on a child's knowledge from where they are in their current stage of development	Expecting a child to be at the same place or have the same interest as their peers

Asking children who are persistent what they need	Asking children who are persistent why they are not following directions
Identifying and working to understand the unmet needs when children present concerning behavior	Labeling the child and their concerning behavior as the problem

Caregivers can prepare for strength-based conversations by presenting observations that display knowledge about the unique qualities of each individual child. Carefully reflect on your own assumptions about the child and then think carefully about preparing neutral observational notes. Reflect on the following:

- What is the child's age and their present stage of development?
  - *Does my expectation of the child match where they are developmentally?*
- What percentage of time do we see this behavior?
  - *Is it consistent, or does it happen occasionally?*
- What is the environment or precursor of triggered behaviors?
  - *What happens before, during, and after the behavior is observed?*
- What is the duration or frequency of the concerning behavior?
  - *Is the behavior new, or has it been observed over time?*
- What effect do the child's day-to-day behaviors or actions have on their large- and small-group interactions?
  - *Is the behavior similar or different from day to day, and what is its frequency in social interactions?*

There are many ways to assess development. As caregivers, we work with screening tools (see chapter 10 for the difference between screening, assessment, and diagnostic tools). Not all developmental tools are designed to be culturally sensitive. Many tools are based on the deficit model, using language that expresses a negative image of the child. If the tools use language focusing on what the child still needs to learn or has not yet achieved, then it is important to reflect carefully on how you can best approach the screening tool's findings. We want to ensure that we are reporting the presenting behaviors from a strength-based approach.

Bias, Implicit Bias, and Work with Children

We recognize that every one of us has learned attitudes about people who are different from us in some way. This section looks at the effect of bias, especially the unintentional bias that can influence how we support children and families in our programs. Talking about biases may make us feel nervous or self-conscious; however, as professionals working with families and young children, we must be sure to address any and all unfounded biased beliefs we learned as children or as adults. Implicit (unconscious) biases can be expressed in our behaviors and decision-making, and even in how welcoming we are to families. Bias directed at a person or group causes them undue stress and feelings of alienation, which harms them. Yet every code of ethics practiced in human service professions includes a statement to the effect of *Do no harm*.

Understanding bias helps reveal beliefs or experiences that slant our actions. Biased beliefs can be, and often are, detected by the other person, consciously or unconsciously. These unchecked biases interfere with establishing and maintaining authentic and meaningful relationships with a child or family. Spending time exploring our own implicit bias can be uncomfortable, but not exploring our bias can influence how we approach relationships, engagement, challenging behaviors, and referral to services by shifting us into a deficit model. This deficit model leads to unequal expectations for children and can ultimately result in biased treatment. Implicit bias is particularly harmful because it often remains unexamined, resulting in caregivers over-referring children to disability or emotional support services. Dominant cultural assumptions about what early childhood behaviors should look and sound like are very narrow in their approach. We must examine our own assumptions and cultural expectations about physical activity, rule following, independence, collaboration, school readiness, and many other dimensions.

NAEYC states, "It is essential to see and understand your own culture in order to see and understand how the cultures of children and their families influence children's behavior. Only then can you give every child a fair chance to succeed" (Kaiser and Rasminsky 2020). NAEYC's Advancing Equity in Early Childhood Position Statement provides these guiding principles:

- recognizing that "self-awareness, humility, respect, and a willingness to learn are key to becoming a teacher who equitably and effectively supports all children and families"
- developing a strong understanding of culture and diversity
- understanding that "families are the primary context for children's development and learning" (NAEYC 2019)

To learn more about unpacking cultural assumptions in working with young children, consider the following resources.

Read:

- *Antibias Education for Young Children and Ourselves* by Louise Derman-Sparks, Julie Olsen Edwards, and Catherine M. Goins, 2nd ed. (Washington, DC: NAEYC, 2000).
- *The Brilliance of Black Boys: Cultivating School Success in the Early Grades* by Brian L. Wright and Shelly Counsell (New York: Teachers College Press, 2018).
- "Talking with Children about Race and Social Justice" by John Nimmo, *Child Care Exchange*, May/June 2020.
- *What If All the Kids Are White? Anti-bias/Multicultural Education for Young Children and Families* by Louise Derman-Sparks, Patricia G. Ramsey, and Julie Olsen Edwards, 2nd ed. (New York: Teachers College Press, 2011).

Watch:

- Walter Gilliam, "Early Childhood Expulsion and Bias," First Things First Early Childhood Summit 2019, www.youtube.com/watch?v=3YBSs20YX40.

Unpacking Dominant Cultural Narratives

Many cultural assumptions surround young children's behaviors in early childhood environments. In our current social and political context, not every group has the same leverage or power. When one group has more influence or power than others, it is considered the dominant cultural group. The dominant culture's narrative in education is the messaging about education as told by the cultural group who holds power. The following activity is designed to help you use a strength-based approach to unpacking the dominant cultural narrative. Read each question and reflect on your responses.

TABLE 9.3. DOMINANT CULTURAL EXPECTATION: PHYSICAL DEVELOPMENT

www.redleafpress.org/scm/9-1.pdf

Children should be able to sit quietly for learning activities.

QUESTIONS TO ASK YOURSELF	YOUR REFLECTIONS
What views and expectations do I have about learning? What were my own experiences of focus and attention in learning? How do my beliefs affect how I view each child's learning style?	
How can I create a culturally responsive classroom adaptation of active inside learning?	

Questions to engage parents in a strength-based approach:
How does your child enjoy learning?
Where do you see your child fully engaged?

Strength-based changes to make to the classroom or curriculum:

TABLE 9.4. DOMINANT CULTURAL EXPECTATION: COGNITIVE DEVELOPMENT

www.redleafpress.org/scm/9-2.pdf

Cognitive development is the most important domain for school readiness.

QUESTIONS TO ASK YOURSELF	YOUR REFLECTIONS
What views and expectations do I have about what makes children smart? What were my own experiences of what developmental domains are valued? How do my beliefs affect how I document each child's learning?	

How can I document the multiple ways children demonstrate their learning through social, emotional, cognitive, linguistic, and physical experiences?

Questions to engage parents in a strength-based approach:
What are your child's favorite activities?
What does your child teach us through how they interact with the world?

Strength-based changes to make to the classroom or curriculum:

TABLE 9.5. DOMINANT CULTURAL EXPECTATION: SOCIAL DEVELOPMENT

Everything needs to be "fair."	
QUESTIONS TO ASK YOURSELF	**YOUR REFLECTIONS**
What views and expectations do I have about distribution of time and materials in the classroom? What were my own experiences with fairness growing up? What are my beliefs about fairness regarding gender? How do my beliefs affect how I feel about children who need more time and energy than others?	
How can I adjust my teaching practices so that every child receives what they need?	

www.redleafpress.org/scm/9-3.pdf

Questions to engage parents in a strength-based approach:
What does your child need to feel a valued part of our community?
What does your child need from me as a caregiver?

Strength-based changes to make to the classroom or curriculum:

PILLAR FIVE: FAMILY RELATIONSHIPS AND CULTURE

TABLE 9.6. DOMINANT CULTURAL EXPECTATION: EMOTIONAL DEVELOPMENT

Emotions should not be messy.

QUESTIONS TO ASK YOURSELF	YOUR REFLECTIONS
What views do I have about strong or big emotions? How was I taught to handle big emotions? How does my comfort with children's big emotions affect my engagement with them?	
How can I develop strategies for honoring all children's emotions?	

Questions to engage parents in a strength-based approach:
How does your family discuss feelings and emotions at home?
What can I do to support your child's emotional health in the classroom?

Strength-based changes to make to the classroom or curriculum:

www.redleafpress.org/scm/9-4.pdf

TABLE 9.7. DOMINATE CULTURAL EXPECTATION: LANGUAGE DEVELOPMENT

Literacy skills are focused on reading and writing.

QUESTIONS TO ASK YOURSELF	YOUR REFLECTIONS
What type of literacy experience did I have as a young child? Do the stories I remember follow a specific story style (beginning, middle, and end), or feature a specific race/ethnicity of hero/villain? How do my own experiences influence how I interpret children's language and literacy development?	

www.redleafpress.org/scm/9-5.pdf

How can I adapt my ideas of language and literacy to recognize how story patterns, language, and literacy development are unique to each culture?

Questions to engage parents in a strength-based approach:
What can you learn about a child's literacy history in the home and their storytelling practices?
How can you incorporate both nonlinear or nontraditional language and literacy styles when working with families?

Strength-based changes to make to the classroom or curriculum:

Final Thoughts

Beginning at birth, young children begin to learn about attitudes, values, preferences, and biases from the people closest to them, including their families and significant caregivers. This learning takes place while the brain is quickly learning and actively restructuring itself. Because everyone learns bias, we believe that it is important for responsive caregivers to reflect on those biases they learned in childhood (or later) that might influence their classroom practice.

Families navigate a complex societal system. Family identity is connected to culture, ethnicity, religion or spiritual beliefs, community, life experiences, and education. Supporting families requires a culturally sensitive, strength-based approach. How we choose to view families and individual children within their family's system significantly affects our relationships with them. Coming to understand how our own experiences and bias influence our classroom interactions is part of the work we do to meet our ethical responsibilities to families.

Taking Action

What Caregivers Can Do

- Understand the family systems of both your own family and the families in your care.

- Learn about different cultural approaches to early childhood development.
- Incorporate different strength-based approaches into your own practices.

Reflection and Application

- How does my own understanding of strength and deficit perspectives affect my engagement with families?
- What work have I done to understand my own implicit bias?
- How do I build strong relationships with families that honor their different ways of knowing?

CHAPTER 10

Pillar Six: Caregiver's Sphere of Influence

Every child deserves a champion—an adult who will never give up on them, who understands the power of connection and insists that they become the best that they can possibly be.
—Rita Pierson

Our work as early childhood caregivers is to support the overall health and wellbeing of young children and help them reach their developmental milestones. But what happens when we have concerns regarding a child's behavior or when children are not meeting their developmental milestones? When faced with challenging situations, responsive caregivers need to ask themselves an important question: *What actions and resources are within my sphere of influence?* We are better able to do the following when we clearly understand our sphere of influence:

- know where ours and others' expertise lies
- understand our role and its strengths and limitations in supporting young children
- recognize the importance of observation, screening, and assessment in children's overall health and wellbeing
- make sound decisions about who and how we refer to services
- explain the broader view of support services that may be available to parents
- incorporate strength-based practices into our care of children

Many additional questions surface as early care providers ponder what is within their sphere of influence and what they can do next to support a child and their family. For example, one of the most difficult tasks for early childhood caregivers is understanding when and where to ask for help and then determining how to incorporate that help into our classroom practice. We ask, *What can I do if I observe developmental delays? Who do I ask for help? What services are available? What classroom strategies can I use, or what training can I take to improve my practice?* These questions and their answers are all part of what we need to know to support children and provide high-quality early care.

The Caregiver's Sphere of Influence

The caregiver's sphere of influence in early care and education is to provide children ages birth through five with high-quality care. Early care and education can be provided in a variety of settings—public and private, profit and nonprofit, faith-based, community-based, home-based, employee-sponsored, tribal, or culturally specific. There are specific programs such as Head Start and Early Head Start, public preschools, and programs influenced by specific pedagogies, such as play-based, Montessori, and Reggio Emilia, to name a few. Individuals working directly with young children—aides, assistant caregivers, caregivers, providers, and directors—provide responsive caregiving. Agencies provide early learning support to caregivers as well as services and compliance structures such as licensing specialists, resource and referral agencies, trainers and professional development supports, and coaches and mentors.

We know that every child deserves quality early care and opportunities to reach their full potential. When we observe children who we believe need to be assessed for more specialized services or interventions, we must take additional steps beyond everyday practice, sometimes including partnering with or referring families to outside support services. In these situations, we are broadening our sphere of influence beyond early learning to connect families with additional support services.

Our work exists within the early care and education field. It also connects to related fields within the larger framework of services and supports for children ages birth to five and their families (see figure 10.1). Within these categories are groups of professionals who provide specialized services. They support caregivers' work in early care and education by providing them additional ways to broaden families' protective factors and assist children and families in receiving needed services. The category of early care and education goes beyond the classroom and includes

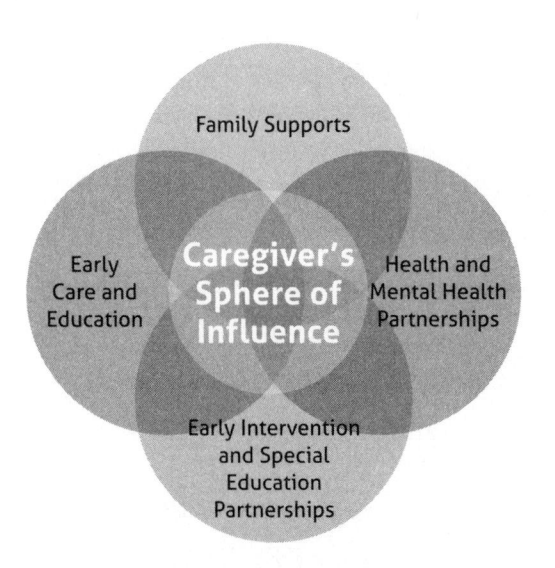

Figure 10.1. Caregiver's Sphere of Influence

educational agencies, services, and professional development, such as school districts, colleges, or NAEYC.

Supporting children and their families is complex work, and many individuals affect children and their families. In quality early care and education, we work to understand how each of these categories intersects with the lives of children, parents, and early childhood caregivers both inside and outside the classroom. Most importantly, we come to recognize our sphere of influence and how we can partner with outside experts in helping children reach their developmental potential.

In this chapter, we look at the first three categories: *family supports*, *health and mental health partnerships*, and *early intervention and special education partnerships*. Professionals in these three categories have specific training and education that prepares them for their role in supporting children, families, and caregivers. See table 2.1, Professional Mental Health Practitioners and Specialists, for a list of professionals and their qualifications. The fourth category is discussed in chapters 11 and 12.

The category of *family supports* focuses on providing supports such as home visiting and structural supports from service organizations. Home visiting is a preventative approach to supporting young children and their families in their home environments, and organizations that undertake home visits include Head Start, Early Head Start, hospitals, and social services agencies, to name a few. Social services come from a wide variety of groups, ranging from local community agencies, food banks, and culturally specific organizations to the federally funded Department of Human Services and Department of Housing and Urban Development. Family supports also include aspects of the legal system, such as courts, foster care, and public safety.

In the *health and mental health partnerships* category, professionals such as doctors, nurses, dentists, and mental health clinicians, among others, provide services to children and their families. The health and mental health fields require formalized education and licensing and ongoing professional development. Pediatric doctors—and increasingly, nurses and nurse practitioners—attend primarily to the physical health and development of young children. They are focused on the physical, behavioral, and mental health of their patients, examining children to ensure that they are developing within a typical range. Pediatric dentists specialize in the care of children's teeth, gums, and mouths and are trained to support young children with disabilities and oral health needs. Mental health clinicians include licensed counselors (infant and toddler, child, and marriage and family) as well as clinical social workers and psychologists who have specialized training in child development, trauma, brain function, and human behavior. They provide supports to address stress and emotional problems, including family or marital issues, grief, depression, anger, and other emotional issues that affect behavior. Psychiatric nurses and psychiatrists address complex emotional and mental health needs, including medical treatment, through drug therapy.

The *early intervention and special education partnerships* category focuses on the supports and services available for young children with a disability or developmental delay. Services are available by law to children who have been diagnosed by a licensed professional, which include early intervention or early childhood special education serving young children in their first three years of life, as well as special education serving youth ages three through twenty-one. Early care programs and schools use two main documents to outline services provided to families who have a child diagnosed with a disability: the Individualized Family Services Plan (IFSP), which covers young children under three years of age, and the Individualized Education Plan (IEP), which applies to children over the age of three. Children with a relevant medical diagnosis can access speech, physical, and occupational therapies, among others. Early intervention and special education offer targeted skill development to help children meet their developmental milestones.

Observation, Screening, and Assessment Practices for Caregivers

As we said earlier, your sphere of influence includes providing high-quality classroom settings that foster children's progression in cognitive, physical, language, and social and emotional development. The caregiver's sphere of influence also includes the practices of observation, screening, and assessment. Caregivers can identify children who seem at risk for developmental delays or exhibit behaviors that could merit further assessment and refer them to specialized professionals.

Observing Development

A significant part of our work as early childhood caregivers is to observe, screen, and assess the overall health and wellbeing of young children, and then use what we learn from our observations, screenings, and assessments to plan developmentally appropriate early learning experiences and respond to children's emotions in developmentally appropriate ways. Our goal is to meet children's cognitive, physical, language, and social and emotional needs through developmentally appropriate practices. Our primary role as caregivers is to use our observations of children to identify and provide what they need to learn and develop so they can grow into their full potential.

Children's development typically follows a logical sequence or continuum. While each child is unique in their development, there are windows of opportunity for optimal development when the body and the brain are aligned to learn specific skills. For example, acquiring motor skills, such as learning to walk and run, typically happens before the age of five. Beginning in infancy, each age range has specific developmental milestones, the skills and competencies that children generally acquire during that period and continue to master over time. Like building blocks, these milestones form the foundation for the next set of developmental skills and competencies. Within each major domain, developmental milestones are identified along an age-related continuum. Observation, screening, and assessment help providers and specialized professionals plan strategies and interventions to support children in reaching their developmental milestones. They are also essential in helping caretaking professionals make sound decisions about when and how to refer children and families to specialists, and to whom.

Asking for help from outside experts when needed is important. Our work is to support children by providing experiences through activities and interactions that help them meet their developmental milestones. When children meet their developmental milestones, it is like they are walking through an open door. When they miss their milestones, it is like pushing a 10,000-pound door open. We observe children to ensure they are developmentally on track in all areas of development. When they are not reaching milestones or progressing along the developmental continuum, we need to refer their families to specialized services and professionals. We want children to reach their developmental milestones within their optimal windows of opportunity. Therefore, timely referrals are critical so children and families receive the support they need as early as possible.

Observational Notes

Before we make any decisions about referring children for additional support services, we need to document what we observe. We know that diagnosing is not within our sphere of influence, but supporting professionals with our observational notes can assist them in their diagnostic process. In chapter 7, we discuss how behaviors need to be observed over time and in multiple settings for diagnostic purposes. Therefore, observational notes are fundamental to any discussion about a child's development or behavior. This is especially important if you have concerns about children's behaviors. Taking observational notes requires a specific set of practices. Here are a few tips to help you accurately capture what you observe:

> Let's use our observations of Ava from chapter 6.
> - When observing the child or children, record *only* what you see.
>   - *Ava is stacking the blocks.*
> - Take care *not* to add any interpretation of what you see.
>   - *Ava is <u>happy</u> stacking the blocks* is an interpretation of Ava's feelings. Instead, write, *Ava is carefully placing one block on top of the other. She stacks a tower of blocks together.*
> - Choose neutral language—do not use feeling words.
>   - *Ava is <u>frustrated</u> when the tower falls down* is not neutral. Instead, write, *Ava throws a block when the tower falls down.*
> - Include the context of what is happening at the time of the observation.
>   - *Ava is working in the block area during morning exploration. The block area is busy with four children building in the space. Ava is working alone while the other three children are working together.*
> - Include basic information about the child or children.

> - *Ava is 3.5 years old, and English is not her primary language. She is an only child. This is her sixth month in our classroom.*
>
> Observation example: *Today is February 12 at 10:26 a.m. Ava is 3.5 years old. English is not her primary language. She is an only child. This is her sixth month in our classroom. Ava is working in the block area during morning exploration. The block area is busy with four children building in the space. Ava is working alone while the other three children are working together. Ava is stacking the blocks. Ava is carefully placing one block on top of the other to create a tower of blocks. When the blocks fall, Ava throws a block.*

Screening and Assessment within the Sphere of Influence

In high-quality programs, early childhood providers are trained to use a variety of screening and assessment tools. These tools help us determine next steps in providing high-quality care, appropriate family support, and early interventions for the children we serve. One screening tool is the Ages and Stages Questionnaire (ASQ-3), which screens children from one month through 5.5 years of age. This strength-based tool is recommended by many of the leading national professional organizations, such as the American Academy of Pediatrics, the American Academy of Neurology, and First Signs.

In settings such as Head Start, the ASQ-3 is used as a valid, reliable, accurate, and cost-effective tool to identify delays in children's development. The ASQ-3 is used by parents, caregivers, and health care professionals alike to identify whether children are meeting their developmental milestones. This screening tool is easy to use and can be completed by parents in a short period of time. It teaches parents about child development and encourages them to be involved in their child's development. It is designed to identify early developmental delays and children who may be at risk for them. If you identify developmental delays or indicative symptoms, you should refer the child's family to specialized services following your program's procedures.

Assessment tools typically require specific training. There are several nationally recognized assessment tools used to evaluate children, classroom environments, and caregiver interactions. They go from simple to complex and require varied types of training and education to administer.

The environmental assessment tools rate the classroom environment, including space and furnishings, personal care routines, listening and talking, program activities, health and safety of the environment, and overall warmth and interactions of caregivers (Environmental Rating Scale 2020). Here are the most widely used environmental rating tools used in our field:

- The Infant/Toddler Environment Rating Scale (ITERS-3) assesses group programs for children birth to age three.
- The Early Childhood Environment Rating Scale (ECERS-3) assesses group programs for children ages three to five years.
- The Family Child Care Environment Rating Scale-3 (FCCERS-3) rates group programming in family child care settings.

The Classroom Assessment Scoring System (CLASS) assessment tool is a valid and reliable instrument that scores the interactions between teacher and student in infant through preschool classrooms. The scoring criteria varies between age groups, beginning with responsive caregiving in infant care. Moving upward in complexity, toddler care is assessed in the domains of emotional and behavioral support and engaged support for learning. In preschool early learning environments, the CLASS instrument expands its criteria to include emotional support, classroom organization, and instructional support (Teachstone 2020).

Being knowledgeable about the different screening and assessment tools helps us better understand our sphere of influence when working with young children. These tools provide us with information to improve our classroom environments and interactions with young children.

Final Thoughts

As early childhood caregivers, we must know and understand our sphere of influence is important. We demonstrate our professional practices by clearly understanding our role and sphere of influence in supporting the overall mental health and wellbeing of young children. We integrate observation, screening, and assessment into our practice and share with parents and experts our understanding of how children are progressing toward their developmental milestones. Our ability to make sound decisions in how we refer to services is also part of our work. We become familiar with the services provided by outside agencies in the areas of family supports, health and mental health, and early intervention and special education. (When referring families to outside support services, make sure those agencies have the availability and currently provide services to help the child and their family.) We offer families a warm handoff by keeping accurate records and making sure the agency's contact information (phone number, address, services, website, and so forth) is still current. One way we do this is by partnering and building relationships with support service agencies and understanding how they work. Many families fall through the cracks or fail to take next steps in receiving the help they need because they find the transfer of care too overwhelming or discover that agencies are no longer offering certain services. Therefore, our careful referrals provide an additional protective factor for families, helping assure that they connect with the specialized services they need.

Taking Action

What Caregivers Can Do

- Establish protocols for support services referrals.
- Check that your agency has up-to-date contacts and scope of services for referral agencies.
- Support parents in contacting agencies by using a warm handoff.
- Become trained in using screening and assessment tools.

Reflection and Application

- How do I see my sphere of influence in supporting children and families?
- How does my sphere of influence foster mental health and wellbeing in young children?
- How do I improve my practice through the use of screening and assessment tools?

SECTION 3

Strength-Based Classroom Strategies

While section 1 of the book introduces mental health and wellbeing, and section 2 focuses on the Six Pillars, section 3 turns toward applying strength-based approaches in classrooms.

- Chapter 11 reviews classroom strategies, the importance of designing strength-based environments to meet children's needs, and curriculum planning, which includes three approaches to strength-based caregiver practices.
- Chapter 12 connects all the themes of the book together and draws conclusions to support strength-based practices for early childhood mental health and wellbeing.

QR Codes and Additional Resources

The QR codes take you to an online section of resources offering materials and practical strategies you can embed in your curriculum and classroom practices, including twenty-five activities focusing on emotional wellness and a list of recommended children's books and internet resources that support social and emotional development.

To access these materials, use the QR code below.

www.redleafpress.org
/scm/11-1.pdf

CHAPTER 11

Strength-Based Classroom Approaches and Resources

Early childhood programs should be places where all children—regardless of family circumstances—can be themselves, with all their feelings, interests, knowledge, and desires.
—Deb Curtis and Margie Carter

We believe that strength-based caregiving lies at the core of the Six Pillars. These approaches help foster children's wellbeing, developing their social and emotional skills and competencies, and building their protective factors to help them face stress or trauma. We have discussed strength-based approaches in detail in chapter 4 and have also woven this approach throughout this book as we've looked closely at the development of children's mental health and wellbeing. The dyadic relationships between a child and their primary caregivers form the foundation of strength-based approaches to responsive care. We believe that loving, nurturing, and responsive caregiving means focusing on the child's positive attributes rather than their deficits. For example, the caregiver recognizes and affirms when children offer to help in the classroom or show empathy and concern when other children are upset or are in distress. By recognizing and affirming these moments, caregivers strengthen children's social and emotional skills and reinforce their willingness to show care and compassion for others. Responsive caregivers focus their interactions on nurturing the whole child and help fulfill the child's unmet needs through strength-based strategies.

Recognizing the individual strengths of children includes honoring their family and cultural backgrounds. Strength-based strategies are grounded in relationships where respectful, nurturing caregivers focus on the existing capacities of children and families. As responsive caregivers, we understand that each child in our care comes to us with their own unique cultural background and life experiences. Families and culture strongly influence the child's developing sense of self and wellbeing. From our family and culture, we learn how to communicate with others, form relationships, and develop beliefs and attitudes toward others. Culture provides children with a rich fund of knowledge about cultural rituals, traditions, and historical perspectives. Our task is to help children build on their current state of wellbeing through a personal caregiving practice that recognizes their individual strengths and looks for the positive qualities in each child. Your early learning environment also plays an important role in promoting children's mental health and wellbeing.

Designing Strength-Based Learning Environments

We believe that responsive caregiving includes both designing early learning environments and planning and implementing curriculum and early learning around strength-based practices. When we are asked how to manage concerning behaviors (often labeled as challenging behaviors) in the classroom, we always first ask the caregiver which strength-based practices they use in their early learning setting. We've seen that integrating strength-based practices into the early care environment prevents or minimizes many behaviors labeled as challenging. We believe that intentional strength-based practices positively influence a classroom's overall culture while also meeting the needs of each individual child. The three approaches outlined in this chapter are meant to assist caregivers in both working with children and families, and planning and designing strength-based early learning environments.

When designing your early learning space, think about how your physical space is organized. Begin by eliminating messy and cluttered areas. When play areas are neat and tidy, children have a sense of predictability and know where materials can be found and where to return them at the end of play. Organized spaces allow for open-ended play, creative expression, and exploration.

We suggest you objectively assess your early learning space in some way. You may use an Environmental Rating Scale (see chapter 10) or other environmental assessment. You may also want to have a trusted colleague, coach, or mentor give you feedback on your overall classroom design. Keep in mind that each group of children requires different strategies and there's no one-size-fits-all answer to designing your strength-based classroom. When planning strength-based classrooms, caregivers design the physical space to accommodate the needs of all children. As you organize and modify your learning space, strive to eliminate any barriers to children's learning. Make modifications throughout the year as children's learning and growing changes.

Caregivers can support children's developing social and emotional development and wellbeing through a variety of design elements, like creating small spaces or cubbies where children can place their personal items. Remember to label childrens' cubbies with their names, as a child's first name is one of the most important words in their vocabulary, and regularly seeing it helps promote their sense of self and self-awareness. Placing children's names in at least three locations around the classroom at their eye level is a good general rule. Also display pictures of the children and their families in areas where children can easily see them, as well as pictures of children engaged in play representing positive social and emotional interactions.

Assess the dominant colors of your learning environment, including walls and furniture. If your walls, display areas, doors, or doorways are finished with bold colors such as bright reds, yellows, and oranges, you may want to redo them. Large areas of bright, bold colors may overstimulate young children's brains. Softer hues or more muted colors similar to those you might find in a natural environment are more relaxing to both children and adults. Highlighting with bright colors here and there is fine, but the overall composition of the classroom color scheme should reflect the calm colors found in nature. Natural materials and low lighting are important too when designing early learning environments.

Most infants and toddlers spend the majority of their exploration time on soft, low furniture or on the floor. Check play areas for glare from overhead lighting and windows by walking through your space during different times of the day and looking at the light both low to the ground and from other angles. Glare on the ceiling or floor may be overstimulating to very young children. Many children are sensitive to fluorescent lights too, so we recommend replacing them with incandescent or LED lights, or lights that have a dimmer switch.

Lastly, think about the noise level in your classroom and how noise can affect the child's sense of wellbeing. Early learning environments are busy and often noisy places where children are learning and growing. As you assess your early learning space, consider both indoor and outdoor noise and how it might disrupt children's learning. If your classroom is near a busy street or next to a parking area full of activity and commotion, consider how you can minimize that outdoor noise or diminish the children's view of outdoor movement. We suggest using window coverings that allow the light to come in or sound reduction machines to minimize outdoor noise and distractions.

Music is a great strength-based tool to use in your classroom. If you want to energize children or transition them from one activity to another, play music with a strong, fast beat, like marching music. If children are being disruptive or not playing well together, listen for the noise level in your learning space. Could noise be overstimulating them and disrupting their thinking and playing? When classrooms become too noisy or disruptive, many teachers choose just to turn off the lights and music. We suggest an alternative strategy: lower the lights and turn on soft instrumental music with a slow, gentle beat. Within a few minutes, you'll observe children's energy and heart rates naturally slowing down. Children will mirror the rhythm of the music as the energy of the classroom lessens. Holistic exercises such as breathing exercises and yoga will help slow the energy level of the classroom as well (see the Mindful Breath and Yoga activities available online).

www.redleafpress.org
/scm/11-2.pdf

Targeted Strength-Based Approaches in the Classroom

Classroom design, curriculum, and planning are important parts of our strength-based practice, but we also know there are times when children need a more targeted approach to prevention. Remember that children desire connection with others, starting with their primary caregivers. When children feel disconnected from adults and peers, they can feel a range of emotions, such as anger, discouragement, frustration, disappointment, and overwhelm. Children who feel disconnected from their primary caregivers also feel unsafe and alone. Young children are rarely able to articulate their needs when they experience these feelings, so they may inadvertently react with behaviors that caregivers find difficult to manage, such as hitting, biting, destroying other children's work, or other disruptive actions. You may also encounter children who have given up trying to get their needs met; these children may lack excitement about trying something new, lack motivation in engaging with others, easily become teary, or remain quiet or withdrawn.

When children demonstrate any of these concerning behaviors, they need immediate, nurturing, and targeted connection with their primary caregivers. If concerning behaviors become more extreme and your classroom activities and approaches are not improving them, it's best to follow your program's policies for referrals for additional support. As you begin to implement these activities, always consider the individual needs of the child and how you can promote their mental health and wellbeing. Also consider your sphere of influence (chapter 10) and how you can best meet the needs of the young children.

The following three approaches will increase your understanding as you work to promote children's mental health and wellbeing. These approaches are not designed to be therapeutic or take the place of work done by licensed mental health professionals.

Approach 1: Using Encouraging Words

The words we use to encourage children are powerful in helping them build and foster their inner feelings of self and personal competencies—their self-identity, self-awareness, confidence, resiliency, and desire to take initiative. Learning the difference between praise and encouragement is important for both parents and early childhood educators (see figure 11.1).

Praise statements are based on the adult's opinion and focus on what the adult thinks and feels, creating short-term positive feelings. Children who are praised too often expect to always hear praise statements from adults and will seek external validation for their efforts rather than develop their own internal motivation. Everyone needs to hear praise now and then. It's wonderful to hear, "You did a great job!" or "What a beautiful picture you painted!" But there is a big difference between praise and encouraging language.

Encouragement helps strengthen the child's own internal messages. Encouragement focuses on the effort of the child and helps them feel proud of their work and accomplishments. It sets children up for success because the adults in their life believe in them and are there to support and encourage them. Statements from adults such as "I believe in you" or "I have confidence that you will make the right decision" are powerful tools in strengthening resolve and resiliency in all children. Encouraging statements help refuel children's self-esteem. We believe in the 20/80 approach: 20 percent praise and 80 percent encouragement.

Wellness Focus

Children hear and learn how to use encouraging language when it is modeled by their caregivers. Children learn to listen to and trust their inner voice. They become persistent when faced with obstacles and develop greater confidence in their abilities.

Exploring Long-Term Resiliency Builders

Don't interrupt children when they are playing. Instead, wait for the closure of play, then refuel their self-esteem by prompting or asking them questions like these:

- Can you share your thinking on this?
- You have important ideas to share. Can you tell me about them?

Short-Term Positive Statements
- I like the way _____ is sitting so quietly.
- I like the way you are playing together.
- I like your _____ (painting).

Long-Term Resiliency Builders
- What's important about your work?
- What was your favorite part?
- What do you like about it?
- What can you tell me about your _____ (picture)?

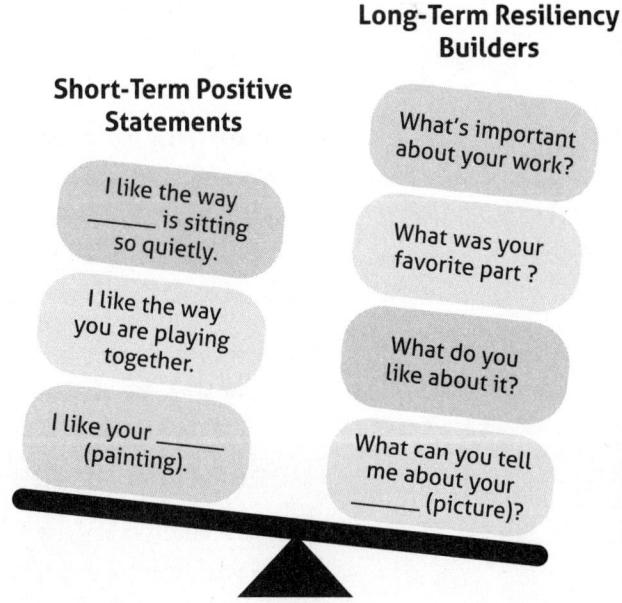

Figure 11.1. Resiliency Builders

STRENGTH-BASED CLASSROOM APPROACHES AND RESOURCES

- What might you want to focus on next?
- What are you thinking about doing next?
- Where do you still have questions?
- What kind of help do you need?
- What helped you make your decisions on building your tower?
- What types of materials did you use, and what do you still need?

Inquiry Questions and Comments

- Reflect on your own feelings as you listen to both praise and encouraging statements.
- Are praise statements about the adult or the child?
- How could a praise statement be rephrased as an encouraging statement?
- How does it feel to you to hear encouraging statements?

Approach 2: Looking behind the Curtain

Because children are still learning how to get their needs met, they often express their needs in unacceptable, challenging, or even dangerous ways. With limited understanding of self-regulation, problem solving, and emotional literacy, children often repeat behavior until they get the results they desire. Unfortunately, this sometimes develops into misguided or challenging habits of behavior.

Caregivers often just see and respond to the outward behavior or emotion—what we call the *curtain*. But to truly understand children's behavior, caregivers must look behind the curtain to consider the goal of the child's behavior and think about how they can use strength-based approaches to assist the child in meeting their needs.

Wellness Focus

Caregivers will gain a deeper understanding of the goals behind children's behavior and consider steps to take that will help meet the child's needs.

Understanding the Goals of Children's Behavior

This is a reflective activity for caregivers to gain a better understanding of the goals behind children's behavior. When working with children (and adults too) ask yourself, *What's the goal of the concerning behavior I'm seeing?* We often see misguided behavior in early care—angry outbursts, hitting, biting, destruction of property, tantrums, or aggression. It's not uncommon also to see attention-seeking behaviors, as well as children who are anxious, fearful, or unwilling to try new things.

Caregivers should review the list below and reflect on the child's behaviors, the adult's response to the child's behaviors, the unmet needs and goals behind the behaviors, and the suggested ways to add strength-based practices and approaches to help meet the needs of each child. In addition, the other activities listed in this chapter and on the website via QR code can help you meet the child's needs and identify the belief behind the child's behavior.

www.redleafpress.org/scm/11-3.pdf

Anger or Aggression

Includes destroying property, hitting, yelling, screaming, throwing objects, etc.

- Adult responses: anger, irritation, reminding, threatening, ignoring, punishing, shaming
- Unmet need/goals behind behavior:
  - "I need to connect with you."
  - "I need to feel a sense of belonging."
  - "I only matter when I get noticed."
  - "I feel powerful when I keep others busy."
  - "Help me, I'm hurting."
  - "Support me in knowing what to do with my anger."
- Strength-based actions:
  - Check your own emotions before responding to children's anger.
  - Scan the environment and make sure the child is safe and has space for movement.
  - Keep your talking to a minimum.
  - Stay within sight while quietly waiting for the child's emotions to start decreasing in intensity.
  - When the child has started to reregulate (color returns to normal, breathing slows and becomes steady), approach them and ask if they want to go into the calm center (see "Cozy and Safe Spaces" on page 167), take a walk, or pursue other activities that allow for movement.

- Find times during the day to engage the child in classroom helper tasks to help them to feel empowered.
- Help the child connect with others through activities that create cooperation, such as group games, parachute play, or other physical activities.

Tantrums

Brief tantrums are common in toddlers. In older children, tantrums include crying spells, screaming, kicking, hitting, stomping feet, rolling on the ground, throwing objects, and so on, and typically stop when the child has achieved their desired goal.

- Adult response: frustration, irritation, yelling, embarrassment, threatening language, giving in to the child's desire for food, treats, extra media time, or postponing naptime or bedtime
- Unmet needs/goals behind behavior:
  - "I need to learn ways to self-regulate."
  - "I need to connect with you."
  - "I need to practice decision-making skills."
  - "Help me learn how to identify my feelings and emotions."
  - "Help me feel like I belong."
  - "Encourage me."
- Strength-based actions:
  - Sit or stay close to the child during their tantrum until they begin to calm down. Keep talking to a minimum. Practice and model deep-breathing techniques.
  - Once they are calmer, ask them if they want to be held or rocked, or if they'd like to hold your hand and go for a walk.
  - When the child is calm, read books about feelings and emotions, color, or play with a persona doll (see below for more information about persona dolls).
  - Help the child practice decision-making skills by offering them realistic choices.
  - Teach emotional literacy skills by reading books about emotions and feelings.
  - Help the child feel a sense of connection and belonging by finding times during the day to encourage them.
  - Help the child build confidence and autonomy by encouraging them to explore new things and develop new skills.

Attention Seeking

Includes interrupting, not following directions, distracting others, etc.

- Adult response: annoyance, irritation, unresponsiveness, ignoring the child
- Unmet needs/goals behind behavior:
  - "I need to connect with you."
  - "I need to feel a sense of belonging."
  - "I need to feel loved."
  - "Help me to know you're trustworthy."
  - "Help me feel seen and heard."
- Strength-based actions:
  - Greet each child by name every morning, and make intentional connections with them throughout the day and at the close of the day.
  - Find opportunities for the child to help, and acknowledge the child's willingness to be a helper.
  - Provide opportunities for the child to partner with other children and develop friendship skills.
  - Help the child practice ways to invite others into play activities.
  - Help the child build confidence and autonomy by encouraging them to explore new things and develop new skills.

Anxiety

Includes anxiety and fear, as well as unwillingness or hesitancy to try new things.

- Adult response: feeling helpless, frustrated, uncertain about how to help
- Unmet needs/goals behind the behavior:
  - "Can I trust you?"
  - "I need you to break directions down into smaller steps."
  - "I need to connect with you; help me feel safe."
  - "I need to feel that someone cares about me."
  - "Help me feel less scared and overwhelmed."
- Strength-based actions:
  - Consider whether the noise level or lighting in the class is over-stimulating to the child, and adjust accordingly.

- Direct the child to a calm area and place items there that the child finds comforting.
- Practice and model deep-breathing techniques.
- Break large- and small-group and transition activities down into smaller steps.
- Help the child practice decision-making skills.
- Find times during the day to encourage and reassure the child that you are there to help them.
- Help the child feel a sense of connection and belonging by finding times during the day to build your relationship with them.
- Help the child build confidence and autonomy by encouraging them to explore new things and develop new skills.

As you work to meet the child's unmet needs behind their curtain, be sure to discuss your concerns with their parents. The more you can partner with parents in supporting the child, the more successful the child will be in developing new social and emotional skills. Be sure to document the concerning behaviors you have observed and the strength-based approaches and activities you have used. As discussed in chapter 7, if concerning behaviors persist and you continue feeling concerned about the child's behavior and development, seek additional support by following your agency's policies for referrals.

Inquiry Questions and Comments

- What concerning behavior is the child exhibiting?
- What do I feel when I see this behavior repeated?
- What do I think is the intended goal of this behavior?
- How do I support the child so they will feel connected and like they belong in our classroom community?
- What social and emotional strengths does the child possess that I can build upon?
- What strength-based strategies have worked in the past?
- What strength-based strategies will I plan to use next?

Approach 3: Using Feeling Words

Young children can struggle to match the emotions in their bodies with the words that describe them. Children need a complex vocabulary to articulate a wide range of emotions. Caregivers help children build their emotional vocabulary as they learn to identify a variety of feeling words.

Convey to children that feelings are neither good nor bad, and that everyone experiences different feelings at different times.

In this approach, caregivers model their own complex emotions through emotional literacy. Be sure to pay attention to how you explain your own feeling words to children. Consider the words *mad*, *angry*, *frustrated*, and *annoyed*. Each word conveys a different level of intensity, from intense to moderate to mild. Word choice in both children and adults gives us insight into a person's self-regulation. Often the stronger the emotions we feel, the simpler the words we use. Using complex words shows that the neocortex's complex reasoning and problem-solving abilities are in place, whereas using simple words indicates that emotions have overwhelmed the neocortex. The difference between *mad* and *annoyed* illustrates this point.

Wellness Focus

Young children need support in expanding their social and emotional vocabulary as they learn that feelings range in intensity from mild to moderate to intense. This strength-based approach not only will help children learn to identify and articulate their own feelings but will also help them in identifying when their emotions are starting to escalate or deescalate as they learn how to self-regulate.

Building an Emotional Vocabulary for Complex Feelings

Building a strong emotional vocabulary works well both in group time and in a dyadic relationship between caregiver and child. We want children to be calm and relaxed when we teach them about emotions. Prepare for the conversation by thinking about all the emotions you feel during the day. Seek images and examples online, such as emotion wheels, charts, and posters, that provide emotional vocabulary words ranging from simple to complex. Emotion wheels go from simple to complex language (mad-frustrated-annoyed or fearful-scared-overwhelmed), supporting children to develop a vocabulary that can identify the nuances of emotions we feel. Select a book that talks about the range of emotions people feel, such as *On Monday When It Rained* by Cherryl Kachenmeister. Then show the emotion wheel, chart, or poster to introduce children to a range of emotions and their corresponding facial expressions.

Begin by discussing simple or mild emotions that children can easily recognize, such as happy, silly, sad, or excited, before talking about more intense feelings, such as fear, frustration, or anger. Help the children to explore simple to complex emotions. Explain to children that feelings are neither good nor bad. Develop a list of words to describe emotions and add to it as children develop their emotional vocabulary. Pass around a hand mirror to help children practice making emotional expressions as you discuss feelings and ask questions such as, "What does *confident* look like?" Don't hesitate to use complex emotions over time; the more words children have to name their emotions, the greater their emotional awareness becomes.

You can come up with your own list of feeling words, but here is a start:

- Brave
- Cheerful
- Bored
- Surprised
- Curious
- Proud
- Disappointed
- Frustrated
- Silly
- Excited
- Uncomfortable
- Fantastic
- Worried
- Friendly
- Loving
- Safe
- Angry
- Generous
- Shy
- Ignored
- Satisfied
- Confident
- Impatient
- Calm
- Embarrassed
- Interested
- Happy
- Peaceful
- Relieved
- Lonely
- Overwhelmed
- Tired
- Confused
- Tense

Inquiry Questions and Comments

What strategies do you use to manage your own range of emotions?
- What are your go-to words, and how can you build on your own vocabulary?
- What feelings arise for you when working with children?
- Are the children struggling with their emotional vocabulary?

- How are you planning to incorporate new words to build emotional literacy?

These three approaches will support you in scaffolding your own strength-based skills. They take time and practice to learn and implement, so spend time reflecting on your practice, especially when your classroom is becoming dysregulated. These three approaches are essential to strength-based caregiving. The more you understand children's behaviors, the better equipped you are to help children build their social and emotional skills and competencies. Scan the QR code to find a variety of online, strength-based activities for children from zero to five years of age that build on these approaches. We suggest you use them as you incorporate strength-based strategies into your curriculum.

www.redleafpress.org/scm/11-4.pdf

Curriculum and Classroom Planning

Young children's activities should be play-based and child-centered, allowing children to express themselves freely as they use their imaginations and creativity in an open and nonjudgmental way. We spoke in detail in chapter 1 about the important role of play in a child's development. When planning, consider how you design your large- and small-group activities, and how they allow you many opportunities to make daily meaningful connections with each child. For example, circle time allows children group opportunities to sing songs, listen to stories, and engage in the learning process. Large group times allow children to learn discrete social and emotional skills, such as listening while others are talking and raising a hand to ask questions. Group activities also allow children to share their thoughts and feelings, listen, and follow directions. Small-group activities provide more focused time between the caregiver and children, usually about three to four children at a time. Smaller group sizes allow more personalized instruction where caregivers can focus on the children's individual needs to help them move forward along the developmental continuum.

Emotional literacy is the cornerstone of strength-based learning and development. Emotional literacy is our ability to recognize not only our own emotions but also the emotions of others. These skills strengthen children's capacity to form relationships and identify and regulate their emotions. Early care providers can promote emotional literacy through a variety of strength-based materials, curricula, and design strategies.

Activities and Materials

Providing books throughout your classroom offers opportunities to teach children social and emotional skills, including the wide range of emotions people feel and express. Books teach problem-solving strategies and show how to share and care for others in a fun way. Books can also reinforce classroom expectations such as not hitting or biting and keeping our hands to ourselves. The QR code includes a comprehensive list of children's books about social and emotional development.

Emotional literacy includes learning the vocabulary words that help us articulate our emotions. Through emotional literacy activities that promote vocabulary building, children can learn more than one word to describe their feelings. A child may externally express feelings of anger while inside themselves they may be feeling frustrated, scared, disappointed, or overwhelmed. As we help children learn about the range of feelings and how to identify them, they become better able to communicate their needs and self-regulate their emotions. Children learn that feelings can change in intensity over time and that they may experience more than one feeling at a time. This is what we call mixed emotions, such as during morning drop-off when a child might feel happy and excited to start a new day but also sad to leave their parent (see "A Bucket of Feelings—Mixed Emotions" activity available online). Emotional literacy also includes understanding how facial expressions and body language show how we feel (see "My Feeling Words: My Face Tells a Story" activity available online).

Early care providers can help children develop these skills by focusing on different social and emotional competencies each month. For example, you might plan one month's curriculum around self-awareness. This might include one week spent learning about individual attributes, such as hair color or eye color, another week talking about families, and another week centering around what children like to do, such as play with cars or blocks. Think about how you might rotate the theme of your dramatic play area from kitchen to restaurant to bakery, or to doctor or veterinary office. Each new theme offers endless opportunities for children to build their vocabulary and engage in novel play and social experiences with peers.

Puppets and dolls give children opportunities through play to focus on social and emotional concepts such as feeling sad, sharing, regulating emotions, resolving conflict, playing cooperatively, and being kind

www.redleafpress.org/scm/11-5.pdf

www.redleafpress.org/scm/11-6.pdf

to others. Typically, early care settings have a variety of dolls, including baby dolls and dolls representing different genders, diversities, and special abilities (see "Baby Doll, Baby Doll" activity available online). Attributes such as the name, age, or even gender of dolls may change depending on the children's play situations. For example, one day the doll may be used in the dramatic play area as a "baby sister" and the next day the doll is identified as the "mommy" or the "daddy."

Similar to baby dolls, persona dolls also allow the children to explore feelings and emotions and develop social and emotional competencies. But the identity of persona dolls—name, age, family, likes, and dislikes—remains constant, and they become valued members of the classroom. Classrooms usually have one or more persona dolls. These dolls can be used for all ages of children and should represent the diversity of the classroom. The teacher gives the doll its own identity, including name, age, birth date, family, likes, dislikes, and life experiences so the provider can employ it in storytelling to teach social and emotional skills (see "Baby Doll, Baby Doll" activity available online). For example, if a child has had their feelings hurt, the teacher might bring the persona doll out at circle time. Then the child or teacher can pretend to use the doll to share a story. For example, the teacher might tell about how the doll had their feelings hurt in the past and how it helped to have the offending person apologize to them. Persona dolls are kept in a safe location in the classroom but are always visible to the children. The children can ask the teacher to see the doll or talk with the doll, but the teacher stays close by to make sure the doll is treated like a respected and valued member of the classroom community. Persona dolls promote inclusivity, diversity, and respect for others in strength-based practices.

Open-ended projects document children's growth and thinking processes. Loose parts such as cardboard, twigs, buttons, fabric pieces, and aluminum foil help children learn to move, manipulate, create, and freely express themselves. Consider how you use open-ended materials to enhance children's social and emotional skills and competencies.

We suggest that a strength-based classroom should include a writing table with plenty of materials like markers, crayons, paper, and so on. Keeping writing materials in other areas of the classroom as well provides children additional opportunities to express themselves through writing and drawing. Art materials, including paint, clay, stamps, stickers, scissors, glue, and modeling materials, allow children to develop creativity

www.redleafpress.org/scm/11-7.pdf

www.redleafpress.org/scm/11-8.pdf

and self-expression. Strength-based classrooms set up writing and art in both indoor and outdoor spaces. When children experience open-ended play outdoors, they benefit from the calming elements of nature, like the feeling of soft wind against their faces and the sounds of chirping birds and rustling leaves.

Extended Play Spaces

Strength-based early learning settings honor children's play experiences by providing places in which children can continue their work over multiple days. We know that imagination and play are the business of childhood. Young children are beginning to explore different materials and play experiences, all of which support the development of the whole child. Often caregivers place time limits on how long children can play in certain learning centers in their classroom. We understand that time limits are necessary to allow all children to play in each learning center, but we also know that the act of revisiting work over time is important too. Allowing children to stop work and then revisit it later in the day, the next day, or even a few days later lets children know that we value their work and play. Consider setting up a space in your learning environment that allows children space to continue their work. These play spaces can be designated indoors, outdoors, or both.

By continuing their play experience over time, children can add to and modify their work while they also develop more complex thinking and problem-solving skills, practice decision-making, and use their imagination and creativity. Think about a project or hobby that you enjoy doing, such as scrapbooking, playing the piano, or journaling. How would you feel if someone placed a time limit on your activity or you were asked to stop halfway through completing it? When we cut off children's work or require cleanup of all ongoing work, children hear the message that their work and thinking are less important than a clean classroom.

To respect children's work and allow them time and space to continue creating, we suggest you place simple signage in designated areas so all members of the community, both adults and children, understand the importance of the ongoing work. For example, a sign that reads *Thinking in Progress* or *Under Construction* will alert everyone in the classroom that those children need more time to complete their project.

Children may not return to their work for several days, which is okay because they may still be thinking about how to change or modify their project. Both thinking and doing are part of the creative process. Documenting the completed work and displaying the documentation is important too and supports children in finding closure to a particular project. This strength-based approach using open-ended materials and time to freely create should be part of how we honor children and their work.

Cozy and Safe Spaces

Creating a cozy or safe place also supports the development of social and emotional skills. Learning how to calm down, problem solve, make decisions, cooperatively play, and regulate feelings are only some of the many skills young children are actively learning. Learning social and emotional skills is a large task to ask of young children, and it takes time and maturation. Each day is different, and some days children will manage their feelings with more ease than on other days. The excitement of free-time activities or the chaos of loud classroom noises may cause children to need a cozy or safe area to relax and recharge. These areas are not for punishment, time-out, or restricting a child's engagement in the classroom but rather designated places where a child can feel safe and learn to calm themselves down and self-regulate using the toys and materials kept there. Generally, these areas are located away from loud areas in your learning space. The cozy space in your classroom or home environment helps children practice self-regulation strategies such as taking calming breaths, reading a book, scribbling or drawing on paper, or looking at problems to find positive solutions. Some cozy areas include noise-canceling headphones for listening to calming music or books on tape or softening the surrounding noise. If space permits, secure see-through netting above the space to make it cozier without blocking caregivers from full view of the children.

Place items inside that you feel the children will enjoy while helping them learn to manage their emotions. Several calming kits are available online that you can use in a cozy place, or you can ask your children what they think might be fun to add. Keep in mind that these items need to be durable. You may want to laminate posters and other items that could become dog-eared or torn. Here are some items you can place in a cozy area:

- a variety of books, including social and emotional books (see appendix A)

- sensory toys such as soft balls, stuffed animals, fidget toys, and stress balls
- sand timer (for visual calming, not for time-out)
- visual posters about emotions and problem-solving techniques
- mirror(s)
- beanbag pillows or soft pillows
- pinwheels for blowing on
- sensory bottles or squeeze bottles
- colorful glitter bottles or snow globes
- bubbles
- baby dolls
- crayons, colored markers, and paper

Introduce your cozy area as you would introduce any other space in your classroom. Children need to learn the expectations for playing and exploring in this space just as they do other areas in your early learning environment. We suggest talking to the children about big emotions like anger, sadness, frustration, and hurt feelings, and how they happen to all of us, then explaining the area's purpose and how it can help them when they are feeling these big emotions. In a large group setting, discuss some of the items from your cozy space, such as baby dolls, an emotion-face chart, or a problem-solving poster. Pass the items around so all the children can see and feel them. Explain how they can use the materials, what your expectations are for children in the area, and how they should clean up when they leave the space. You may want to repeat this discussion over a few days so the children will fully understand how to use the space. We suggest that you ask children for suggestions of materials or objects to add to the space as you design your cozy area to promote their interest in and buy-in for the cozy space. At first, invite children to explore the books, soft materials, and posters you have placed there. Over time they will independently explore this space like they do other areas of your early learning environment.

As we said earlier, a cozy area or space is not for punishment, nor does it reward misbehavior. The purpose of the cozy space is to promote children's wellbeing and help them feel safe and learn how to relax and calm their emotions. It's up to you to decide how many children can be in the cozy space at one time. Some children may prefer to be in the space alone, while others may wish for a friend to join them. You may want to keep this decision flexible depending on the child and the kind of emotions they are exhibiting. Knowing your children well will help you make this decision.

When children are experiencing big emotions such as anger or rage, it's best for only the child and possibly an adult to be in the area, as being left alone there may be too much for a child who becomes easily frustrated, angry, or overwhelmed. In these situations, we believe children need one-on-one attention from a responsive caregiver. To feel safe and calm, children need connections with loving caregivers. Sometimes your positive connection with the child can help you invite them into the cozy space before their emotions intensify; sometimes they just need to feel your presence near them to regain their sense of composure. We suggest you sit near the child and practice slowing down your own breathing, then doing a self-check to see what nonverbal messages you might be sending. Children are quick to respond to our tone of voice and body language, which can easily escalate or deescalate the child's behavior.

Children who mistreat or abuse the materials in the cozy space need to be reminded of the area's purpose. If you see this behavior, we suggest going over the purpose and expectations of the cozy space again with the entire class without singling out individual children.

Transitions and Routines

Responsive planning also encompasses the routines and transitions that provide structure and predictability to your classroom. Routines diminish children's anxiety and help them feel safe, secure, and at ease in your early care setting. They provide children with a sense of security about what is going to happen next. Children rely on what they already know about the environment as they transition to new activities. For example, as a child transitions to the outdoor space, they know where the tricycles are and where to return them. Daily routines may include arrival and departure, eating, napping, handwashing, diapering or toileting, free-choice time, and circle time or story time. Along with routines, transitions help children learn how to think about moving (mentally sequencing) from one activity to another. Transitions occur throughout the day as children go from one activity to another, such as moving from whole group time to free time or from outdoor play to indoors and handwashing. Because children often have to wait during these times, they can become wiggly and impatient, so plan regular transition activities such as a song, finger

www.redleafpress.org
/scm/11-9.pdf

www.redleafpress.org
/scm/11-10.pdf

www.redleafpress.org
/scm/11-11.pdf

www.redleafpress.org
/scm/11-12.pdf

play, or game to let children know they are moving from one activity or learning space to another.

Look for everyday opportunities to implement strength-based activities into routines and transitions. For example, take a few minutes every day to incorporate yoga into your routine (see "Yoga: Our Jungle Adventure" activity available online). Taking a mindful walk outdoors offers children opportunities to become more aware of the sights and sounds of nature (see "Mindful Breath Activity: Circle Walking" available online). As you include strength-based activities in your routines, also seek ways to partner with families by asking parents to practice strength-based learning to further support the wellbeing of the child. Use the online activities, such as social stories (see "'I Am . . .' A Social Story") or the emotion wheel (see "My Feeling Words: My Face Tells a Story"), to extend this home/school connection. Consider stocking a lending library for families or providing them a list of recommended social and emotional books.

Create classroom routines such as a morning welcome song or a special way to say goodbye at the end of the day. Hello routines start the day by making the children feel welcome into your care. A warm goodbye, such as, "Good-bye, Juan, it was fun having you in class today. I look forward to seeing you tomorrow!" helps children feel nurtured while providing them with a positive closure to their day in your care. Children who may have had a few tears or upset feelings that day can leave on an encouraging note knowing that their caregiver is looking forward to seeing them the next day. For some children, the early learning environment may be one of the only places where they feel safe, and therefore providing routines, transitions, and loving care in your classroom helps promote that child's feelings of love, safety, and belonging.

Final Thoughts

Your early learning environment plays an important role in helping to meet the learning and developmental needs of each child. How you plan your classroom and implement learning strategies is essential to the children's mental health and wellbeing. When planning your classroom and strength-based activities, always consider the Six Pillars of your sphere of influence—if you see or hear anything that concerns you about the child's safety and wellbeing, take steps to follow your agency's policies.

Many caregivers view children's behavior from a deficit model rather than a strength-based one by labeling some children as *challenging*. These children may feel frustrated or discouraged or lack the social and emotional skills they need to self-regulate or manage their feelings. Remember that children need to emotionally connect with others to feel a sense of belonging. We believe that a strength-based approach to classroom design, curriculum, and planning will help you transform your early learning environment's culture into one of strength and positivity, where children feel loved, nurtured, connected, encouraged, and valued so they can develop the skills they need to manage difficult situations and changes in their lives. Consider the needs of all the children in your care as you design or modify your learning environment, for each child is unique in how they learn and develop and where they are on the developmental continuum. The knowledge and skills you bring to your interactions with children create the culture of your early care setting, and how you design and implement your early learning environment to meet each child's unique needs will strongly influence their mental health and wellbeing. The provided online activities offer a variety of strength-based approaches to further support your strength-based early learning setting.

Taking Action

What Caregivers Can Do

- Assess the classroom for strength-based approaches and review the twenty-five additional activities using the QR code.
- Identify books and materials that support social and emotional development.
- Create a cozy space or corner in your classroom.

Reflection and Application

- How can I share with my colleagues what I know about strength-based practices?
- Design a model for a strength-based classroom and find ways to share it with your colleagues.
- Create a community around strength-based practices in which providers can share new ideas.

CHAPTER 12

Becoming a Strength-Based Caregiver

Make sure the message of love and respect gets through. Start with "I care about you. I am concerned about this situation. Will you work with me on a solution?"
—Jane Nelsen

Throughout this book we have approached supporting children's mental health and wellbeing through the Six Pillars of strength-based caregiving. The framework of the Six Pillars is set around understanding children's social and emotional development; nurturing the dyadic relationship and the children's attachment to their primary caregivers; understanding concerning behaviors; considering factors that impact a child's risk and resiliency; celebrating the role that family relationships and culture play on the child's development; and knowing your role as a responsive caregiver and your sphere of influence.

We know that early care providers support the Six Pillars by providing high-quality responsive care that includes strength-based approaches and practices. Responsive, nurturing caregiving is the foundation for quality early care and the development of children's social and emotional skills, competencies, mental health, and wellbeing. These skills develop along a continuum beginning in infancy, when early attachments to primary caregivers are essential and set young children on a trajectory to developing feelings of safety, security, trust, and resiliency. How children learn to think, solve problems, develop friendships, make decisions, and regulate emotions all begin developing during their early years.

During the first five years of life, young children are actively learning and exploring the world. During this period, their brains are rapidly developing as they build important neurological pathways. They are learning many things along the developmental continuum, including important social and emotional skills. This includes how to recognize not only their own feelings and emotions but those of their caregivers and peers, as well as follow directions, communicate, and regulate their emotions. Also during the first five years of life, children are learning to share, play cooperatively, express empathy and compassion, and more. Nurturing and responsive early care is critical to the child's overall brain development, including their mental health and sense of wellbeing. We believe that strength-based approaches provide caregivers with the knowledge, classroom tools, and strategies to meet the individual needs of the developing child. Respecting the unique qualities each child brings to the setting allows providers to design meaningful experiences to promote children's mental health and wellbeing.

In chapter 8, we discussed risk and resiliency and how to support children who may be at risk or have been exposed to trauma. Developing children's social and emotional skills and competencies through strength-based approaches to caregiving lessens their risk factors and promotes their resiliency to adverse childhood experiences and life's changing situations, including stress and trauma. We understand that we can't prevent children from being exposed to challenging circumstances in life, but we can provide them with loving, nurturing, responsive care that will better equip them to handle whatever they encounter. Understanding your sphere of influence will help you when you become concerned about children who may be at risk or children who exhibit challenging behavior or who are not meeting their developmental milestones.

Strength-Based Strategies

The Six Pillars provide us with a framework to enhance our caregiving and strengthen the quality of care we provide to foster children's mental health and wellbeing. Strength-based approaches are developed through nurturing and caring dyadic relationships and thoughtful and intentional play-based activities. We discussed many strength-based strategies and approaches throughout this book as we've looked closely at the development of children's mental health and wellbeing. We believe that children develop their sense of security, trust, and safety when providers use strength-based approaches to design developmentally appropriate classroom activities. As you plan play-based activities, consider how you use observation and assessment to document children's growth along the developmental continuum, and reflect on how you can use this information in your classroom planning.

How you design your classroom helps foster children's social and emotional development. Creating a safe or cozy corner is an easy way to promote children's ability to regulate their emotions and feel safe and relaxed in your care. We provide an extensive list of age-appropriate social and emotional books (see appendix A) covering a wide range of relevant topics that can be used in both large- and small-group discussions with children in the classroom to promote social and emotional development and a sense of wellbeing. The strength-based activities and approaches in chapters 11 and the twenty-five activities linked to the QR code can be adapted and modified to meet the needs of the children in your care.

As responsive caregivers, we understand that each child in our care comes to us with their own background and experiences. Each family and culture provides children with rich experiences, personal values, family rituals, and traditions that are part of the individuality of each child. Our task as care providers is to respect and honor each child and build on the family's cultural values and beliefs to positively influence a child's mental health and wellbeing. Likewise, each child comes to us with their own set of strengths and needs. There's no one-size-fits-all approach to caregiving. When we observe children's behaviors, we must look at both their met and unmet needs. Challenging classroom behaviors must be seen as outward expressions of unmet needs, and as we work with young children, we must use this approach to learn how to change our reactions and beliefs about those behaviors.

A strength-based approach looks behind the curtain to begin to identify the underlying issues facing the child and their needs. Only then can we begin to plan classroom strategies to help mitigate the child's needs and positively influence the child's mental health and wellbeing.

A strength-based approach to caregiving recognizes and builds on the child's current state of wellbeing through a personal caregiving practice that recognizes their strengths and looks for the positive in them. Strength-based early care settings equip children with the skills and competencies needed to promote feelings of self-confidence, safety, security, and trust—skills that promote resiliency and a positive, hopeful outlook on life. The early years form the foundation of how children will express their feelings, form relationships, and learn throughout their lifetime.

Commit Yourself to Strength-Based Practices

Again, we congratulate you for exploring the many factors that influence the mental health and wellbeing of young children. We hope you have come away with a deeper understanding of the complexities of mental health and wellbeing. Recognizing that there is a large range of mental health disorders and that mental illness and mental health are two separate dimensions will help you as you evaluate when referrals to outside professionals are needed. We suggest you keep an updated list of outside early childhood professionals (see table 2.1) and their current information.

Who you are as a caregiver is as important to the wellbeing of the children in your care as the curriculum you provide for them. What you bring to the dyadic relationship is essential to the development of the child's mental health and wellbeing. Understanding the changing needs of each child in your care can be a daunting task, but establishing a strength-based approach creates a learning environment based on children's strengths rather than their deficits. Your own self-care is important too in providing quality early care, as is understanding your sphere of influence. We hope you will continue to follow your interest and personal journey in strength-based approaches as you promote children's mental health and wellbeing.

Final Thoughts

The care and wellbeing of young children is an awesome responsibility for caregivers. Your role is understanding the complexity of the developing child and how strength-based approaches can set them on a path toward positive relationships and feelings of self-confidence, safety, security, and trust. We hope that every child has the opportunity to be cared for in a setting where they feel loved and can thrive. Helping children learn to become respectful, trustworthy, and capable human beings is a gift you give all of us. Recognizing the limitless potential of each child provides them with a positive outlook on life. Your gift of compassion and care to our youngest children will last them a lifetime.

Taking Action

What Caregivers Can Do

- Explore the strength-based approaches presented in this book.
- Learn more about the cultural backgrounds of the children in your care.
- Read books and articles and listen to podcasts about strength-based approaches.
- Begin a dialogue with colleagues about best practices of quality care.

Reflection and Application

- What are my beliefs about the children in my care?
- How can I change my classroom practices so that I utilize more strength-based approaches?
- How do I support my own emotional health so I can consistently provide responsive care?

APPENDIX A

Recommended Children's Books for Social and Emotional Development

* indicates a board book

BOLD indicates inclusion in the Online Activities

A New School by Kirsten Hall

A Splendid Friend, Indeed by Suzanne Bloom

Abuela's Weave by Omar S. Castañeda

Alphabreaths: The ABCs of Mindful Breathing by Christopher Willard

Baby Faces by Margaret Miller*

Baby Touch and Feel: Animals by Dawn Sirett*

Balancing Act by Ellen Stoll Walsh

Barnyard Dance! by Sandra Boynton

Be Positive: A Book about Optimism by Cheri Meiners

Be Who You Are by Todd Parr

Bear Can't Wait by Karma Wilson

Bear Says Thanks by Karma Wilson

Bear's Busy Family by Stella Blackstone

Bread, Bread, Bread by Ann Morris

Breathe with Me: Using Breath to Feel Strong, Calm and Happy by Mariam Gates

Breathing Makes It Better by **Christopher Willard and Wendy O'Leary**

Brown Bear, Brown Bear, What Do You See? by Bill Martin Jr. and Eric Carle*

Busy! by Annie Kubler*

Charlotte and the Quiet Place by Deborah Sosin

Clap Hands by Helen Oxenbury*

Daddy and Me by Tiya Hall*

Daddy Kisses by Anne Gutman*

Dancing Feet! by Lindsey Craig

Diez deditos de las manos y Diez deditos de los pies / Ten Little Fingers and Ten Little Toes by Mem Fox*

Dino Parade by Thom Wiley

Dinosaurumpus! by **Tony Mitton**

Don't Touch, It's Hot by **David Algrim**

Dreamers by Yuyi Morales

Duck and Goose by Tad Hills*

Duck & Goose, How Are You Feeling? by **Tad Hills***

Everywhere Babies by Susan Meyers*

Eyes, Nose, Fingers, and Toes: A First Book about You by Judy Hindley

Friends at School by Rochelle Bunnett

From Head to Toe by Eric Carle*

Giraffes Can't Dance by Giles Andreae*

Glad Monster, Sad Monster by Anne Miranda

Go! Go! Go! Stop! By Charise Mericle Harper*

Goose Needs a Hug by **Tad Hills***

Hats (Talk-About-Book) by Debbie Bailey

Heartprints by P.K. Hallinan*

Heather Has Two Mommies by Lesléa Newman

Heroines and Heroes / Heroinas y Heroes by Eric Hoffman

How Do Dinosaurs Play with Their Friends? by **Jane Yolen***

How Do Dinosaurs Say I Love You? by Jane Yolen

How Do Dinosaurs Say I'm Mad? by Jane Yolen

How Do I Love You? by **Marion Dane Bauer***

How the Crayons Saved the Rainbow by **Monica Sweeney**

How to Be a Friend: A Guide to Making Friends and Keeping Them by **Laurie Krasney Brown and Marc Brown**

Hug by Jez Albourough*

I Like Me! by Nancy Carlson

I Love You, Daddy by Jillian Harker

177

I Went Walking by Sue Williams*

I'm Happy-Sad Today by Lory Britain

I'm Sorry by Sam McBratney

I'm Thankful Each Day by P.K. Hallinan*

If You Give a Mouse a Cookie by Laura Numeroff

It's Okay to Be Different by Todd Parr

It's Okay to Make Mistakes by Todd Parr

Join In and Play by Cheri J. Meiners

Listen and Learn by Cheri J. Meiners

Listening Time by Elizabeth Verdick*

Listening with My Heart: A Story of Kindness and Self-Compassion by Gabi Garcia

Little Teddy Bear's Happy Face Sad Face by Lynn Offerman*

Lizzy's Ups and Downs by Jessica Harper

Lots of Feelings by Shelley Rotner

Mommy Hugs by Anne Gutman and Georg Hallensleben*

Mommy, Mama and Me by Lesléa Newman*

Mommy's Little Star by Janet Bingham

My First Body by DK Publishing*

My Five Senses by Aliki

My Hands by Aliki

My Heart Fills with Happiness by Monique Gray Smith

My Magic Breath: Finding Calm through Mindful Breathing by Nick Ortner

My Very First Book of Food by Eric Carle*

Noisy Animals by Libby Walden and Tiger Tales*

On Monday When It Rained by Cherryl Kachenmeister

One Duck Stuck by Phyllis Root

Only One You / Nadie Como Tu by Linda Kranz

Planting a Rainbow by Lois Ehlert*

Reach / Alcanzar by Elizabeth Verdick*

Red: A Crayon's Story by Michael Hall

Rumble in the Jungle by Giles Andreae

Sharing Time by Elizabeth Verdick*

Sometimes When I'm Mad by Deborah Serani

Swimmy by Leo Lionni

Ten Little Fingers by Annie Kubler

That's What a Friend Is by P.K. Hallinan*

The Day You Begin. Jacqueline Woodson

The Don't Worry Book by Todd Parr

The Feelings Book by Todd Parr*

The Grouchy Ladybug by Eric Carle*

The Joyful Book by Todd Parr

The Kissing Hand by Audrey Penn

The Rainbow Fish by Marcus and J. Alison James

The Way I Feel by Janan Cain

Today I Feel Silly: And Other Moods That Make My Day by Jamie Lee Curtis

Too Loud Lily / Lily La Ruidosa by Sofie Laguna

Try-Again Time by Elizabeth Verdick*

Two Eyes, a Nose, and a Mouth by Roberta Grobel Intrater

We Are All Alike . . . We Are All Different by Cheltenham Elementary School Kindergartners

We Are Best Friends by Aliki

We Listen to Our Bodies by Lydia Bowers

When I Care about Others by Cornelia Maude Spelman

When I Feel Afraid by Cheri Meiners

When I Miss You by Cornelia Maude Spelman

When Sophie's Feelings Are Really, Really Hurt by Molly Bang

Where Will I Live? by Rosemary McCarney

Wiggle by Doreen Cronin

Yoga Bear: Simple Poses for Little Ones by Sarah Jane Hinder*

Yoga Bug: Simple Poses for Little Ones by Sarah Jane Hinder*

Yoga Whale: Simple Poses for Little Ones by Sarah Jane Hinder*

You Be You / Sé Siempre Tú by Linda Kranz

APPENDIX B

Websites and Internet Resources

ACEs Aware
www.acesaware.org

ACEs Aware is an initiative lead by the Office of the California Surgeon General and the Department of Health Care Services to bring awareness to the lifelong impact of Adverse Childhood Experiences (ACEs). This initiative includes partnering with other organizations to bring awareness and include training, tools, screening, and other resources that promote the health and wellbeing of individuals and families.

Anti-Bias Leaders in Early Childhood Education: A Guide to Change
www.antibiasleadersece.com

Anti-Bias Leaders in Early Childhood Education includes resource guides, films, and professional development focused on anti-bias work in ECE classrooms, demonstrating the importance of teacher reflection on identity, context, and practice in anti-bias education.

The Center on the Developing Child—Harvard University
www.developingchild.harvard.edu

The Center on the Developing Child is a research and development platform working around the world by creating science-based, innovation-friendly environments in which practitioners, researchers, policymakers, and investors can come together to test new ideas, engage in active learning, and solve complex problems to improve outcomes for children.

Center on the Social and Emotional Foundations for Early Learning (CSEFEL)
www.cesefel.vanderbilt.edu

CSEFEL is focused on promoting social-emotional development and school readiness in young children ages birth through five. It provides resources and evidence-based practices that support early education professionals in integrating social-emotional development into their practice. It provides user-friendly materials, videos, and other resources for families and early childhood trainers, coaches, teachers, and caregivers. Materials are offered in English and Spanish.

The Discovery Source
thediscoverysource.com

The Discovery Source creates innovative, effective, and affordable solutions to meet the unique opportunities and challenges that come with nurturing the social-emotional and cognitive development of young learners. This organization has a variety of social-emotional tools offered in English and Spanish, including calming kits, to promote social-emotional development in young learners.

The National Association for the Education of Young Children (NAEYC)
www.naeyc.org

NAEYC is the leading organization for those working with and advocating on behalf of children from birth to age eight. This website offers information about the association and its efforts to support early childhood education professionals, including educational resources, current research, requirements for program accreditation, information on developmentally appropriate practices, public policy issues, and relevant publications.

National Alliance on Mental Illness (NAMI)
www.nami.org

NAMI provides education, support, public awareness, and advocacy for individuals and families who are affected by mental illness. NAMI's goal is to provide education across the United States to people affected by mental illness to help them live healthy and fulfilling lives.

Possibilities ECE
www.possibilitiesece.com

Possibilities ECE supports early childhood educators focused on reflective professional practices by offering affordable workshops in strength-based approaches to early childhood practices. Possibilities ECE publishes a blog centered on building community through early childhood education's work in classrooms, programs, and society.

Search Institute
www.search-institute.org

Search Institute partners with organizations to conduct and apply research that promotes positive youth development and advances equity. It offers free downloadable resources on developmental assets. Search Institute works with schools, family programs, and youth programs and coalitions.

Teaching Tolerance
www.tolerance.org

Part of the Southern Poverty Law Center, Teaching Tolerance provides resources for anti-bias issues and topics. Look for free teacher resources, including curriculum and a weekly newsletter.

Zero to Three National Center for Infants, Toddlers, and Families
www.zerotothree.org

This organization informs, trains, and supports professionals, policy makers, and parents who are working to improve the lives of infants and toddlers. Free blogs and resources are available on the site. Memberships and workshops are also available.

REFERENCES

ACES Aware. 2020. "The Science of Trauma Fact Sheet." Last modified February 25. www.acesaware.org/wp-content/uploads/2019/11/ACEs-Aware-Science-of-Trauma-Fact-Sheet-2-25-20-FINAL.pdf.

Administration for Children and Families. 2021. "Preventing Exclusion and Expulsion from Child Care Programs." https://childcare.gov/index.php/consumer-education/preventing-exclusion-and-expulsion-from-child-care-programs.

Ainsworth, Mary D. S. 1978. "The Bowlby-Ainsworth Attachment Theory." *Behavioral and Brain Sciences* 1 (3): 436–38.

Alonso, J., A. Buron, R. Bruffaerts, Y. He, J. Posada-Villa, J. P. Lepine, and World Mental Health Consortium. 2008. Association of Perceived Stigma and Mood and Anxiety Disorders: Results from the World Mental Health Surveys. *Acta Psychiatrica Scandinavica* 118 (4): 305–14.

Attachment and Trauma Treatment Center. 2020. "Understanding and Working with the Window of Tolerance." Accessed December. www.attachment-and-trauma-treatment-centre-for-healing.com/blogs/understanding-and-working-with-the-window-of-tolerance.

Bruner, Jerome. 1985. "Models of the Learner." *Educational Researcher* 14 (6): 5–8.

Carter, Margie, and Deb Curtis. 2015. *Designs for Living and Learning*. 2nd ed. St. Paul, MN: Redleaf Press.

The Center on the Social and Emotional Foundations for Early Learning (ND). 2021. "Research Synthesis - Infant Mental Health and Early Care and Education Providers." Vanderbilt University. Accessed October 1. https://scpitc.org/wp-content/uploads/2019/03/rs_infant_mental_health.pdf.

Centers for Disease Control and Prevention (CDC). 2020a. "Adverse Childhood Experiences." Accessed October. www.cdc.gov/violenceprevention/aces.

———. 2020b. "Autism Prevalence Rises in Communities Monitored by CDC." www.cdc.gov/media/releases/2020/p0326-autism-prevalence-rises.html.

———. 2020c. "What Is Children's Mental Health?" Accessed April. www.cdc.gov/childrensmentalhealth/index.html.

———. 2020d. "Risk and Protective Factors." Accessed October. www.cdc.gov/violenceprevention/childabuseandneglect/riskprotectivefactors.html.

Child Development Institute at University of North Carolina at Chapel Hill. 2020. "Environmental Rating Scale Family of Products." https://ers.fpg.unc.edu/environment-rating-scales.

Children's Bureau. 2014. "Parenting a Child Who Has Experienced Trauma." www.childwelfare.gov/pubPDFs/child-trauma.pdf#:~:text=When%20children%20have%20experienced%20trauma%2C%20particularly%20multiple%20traumatic,adults%2C%20or%20even%20dissociation%20%28feeling%20disconnected%20from%20reality%29.

Day, Jennifer R., and Ruth A. Anderson. 2011. "Compassion Fatigue: An Application of the Concept to Informal Caregivers of Family Members with Dementia." *Nursing Research and Practice* 2011: 408024. doi:10.1155/2011/408024.

Environmental Rating Scale. 2020. https://ers.fpg.unc.edu/development-iters-r%E2%84%A2.

Gilliam, Walter S. 2005. *Prekindergarteners Left Behind: Expulsion Rates in State Prekindergarten Systems*. New York: Foundation for Child Development.

Gilliam, Walter S., and Chin R. Reyes. 2018. "Teacher Decision Factors That Lead to Preschool Expulsion." *Infants & Young Children* 31 (2): 93–108.

Gopalkrishnan, Narayan 2018. "Cultural Diversity and Mental Health, Considerations for Policy and Practice." *Front Public Health* 6:179.

Kaiser, Barbara, and Judy Sklar Rasminsky. 2019. "Valuing Diversity; Nurturing Curiosity." *Teaching Young Children* 13 (2). www.naeyc.org/resources/pubs/tyc/dec2019/valuing-diversity-developing-understanding-behavior.

Katz, Lilian G. 1993. "Turning Kids' Attention Outward Is the Real Key to Self-Esteem." Deseret News. *New York Times*. www.deseret.com/platform/amp/1993/7/25/19057585/turning-kids-attention-outward-is-the-real-key-to-self-esteem.

Lillas, C., and J. Turnbull. 2009. *Infant/Child Mental Health, Early Intervention, and Relationship-Based Therapies: A Neurorelational Framework for Interdisciplinary Practice*. New York: Norton.

Lipscomb, S.T., B. Hatfield, E. Goka-Dubose, H. Lewis, and P.A. Fisher. 2021. "Impacts of Roots of Resilience Professional Development for Early Childhood Teachers on Young Children's Protective Factors." *Early Childhood Research Quarterly* 56: 1–14.

Mental Health America (MHA). 2000. "What Every Child Needs for Good Mental Health." www.mhanational.org/what-every-child-needs-good-mental-health.

National Alliance on Mental Illness (NAMI). 2020a. "Mental Health by the Numbers." Accessed September 20. https://nami.org/mhstats.

———. 2020b. "Risk of Suicide." Accessed September 15. www.nami.org/learn-more/mental-health-conditions/related-conditions/risk-of-suicide.

National Association for the Education of Young Children. 2005. "NAEYC Early Childhood Program Standards." www.naeyc.org/resources/position-statements.

———. 2011. "NAEYC Code of Ethical Conduct and Statement of Commitment." www.naeyc.org/resources/position-statements/ethical-conduct.

———. 2016. "Standing Together against Suspension and Expulsion in Early Childhood: Resources." www.naeyc.org/standing-together-against-suspension-expulsion-early-childhood-resources.

———. 2019. "Advancing Equity in Childhood Education Position Statement." www.naeyc.org/resources/position-statements/equity.

National Child Traumatic Stress Network. www.nctsn.org.

National Children's Alliance. 2020. "National Statistics on Child Abuse." Accessed March 20. www.nationalchildrensalliance.org/media-room/national-statistics-on-child-abuse.

National Scientific Council on the Developing Child. 2004. *Young Children Develop in an Environment of Relationships*. Harvard University, Center on the Developing Child.

Office of Juvenile Justice and Delinquency Prevention. 2000. "Safe from the Start: Taking Action on Children Exposed to Violence." www.ncjrs.gov/pdffiles1/ojjdp/182789.pdf.

Osgood, Jayne. 2012. *Narratives from the Nursery: Negotiating Professional Identity in Early Childhood*. New York: Routledge.

Parten, Mildred B. 1932. "Social Participation among Preschool Children." *Journal of Abnormal and Social Psychology* 27 (3): 243–69. doi:10.1037/h0074524.

Perry, Bruce D. 2020. "Traumatized Children: How Childhood Trauma Influences Brain Development." *Journal of the California Alliance for the Mentally Ill* 11 (1): 48–51 www.aaets.org/traumatic-stress-library/traumatized-children-how-childhood-trauma-influences-brain-development.

Perry, Bruce D., and Maria Szalavitz, 2007. *The Boy Who Was Raised as a Dog: And Other Stories from a Child Psychiatrist's Notebook*. New York: Basic Books.

Piaget, Jean. 1973. *The Child and Reality: Problems of Genetic Psychology.* Translated by Arnold Rosin. New York: Grossman.

Rogoff, Barbara. 2003. *The Cultural Nature of Human Development*. Oxford: Oxford University Press.

Search Institute. 2020a. "Free Resources from Search Institute." Accessed February 20. www.search-institute.org/our-research.

———. 2020b. 40 "Developmental Assets for Early Childhood (ages 3–5)."

Shonkoff, J. P., A. S. Garner, B. S. Siegel, M. I. Dobbins, M. F. Earls, L. McGuinn, and D. L. Wood. 2012. "The Lifelong Effects of Early Childhood Adversity and Toxic Stress." *Pediatrics* 129 (1): 232–46. http://dx.doi.org/10.1542/peds.2011-2663.

Sorte, Joanne, Inge Daeschel, and Carolina Amador. 2017. *Nutrition, Health and Safety for Young Children: Promoting Wellness*, 3rd ed. Upper Saddle River, NJ: Pearson.

Statman-Weil, Katie. 2020. *Trauma-Responsive Strategies for Early Childhood*. St. Paul, MN: Redleaf Press.

Stegelin, Dolores A. 2018. "Preschool Suspension and Expulsion: Defining the Issues." Institute for Child Success. www.instituteforchildsuccess.org/publication/preschool-suspension-and-expulsion-defining-the-issues.

Teachstone. 2020. "Classroom Assessment Scoring System." Accessed February 15. https://teachstone.com/class.

U.S. Department of Justice. 2020. "Safe from the Start: Taking Action on Children Exposed to Violence." www.ojp.gov/pdffiles1/ojjdp/182789.pdf.

Vygotsky, Lev. S. 1980. *Mind in Society: The Development of Higher Psychological Processes*. Cambridge, MA: Harvard University Press.

Whitebread, David. 2017. "Free Play and Children's Mental Health." *Lancet Child & Adolescent Health* 1 (3): 167–69. www.thelancet.com/pdfs/journals/lanchi/PIIS2352-4642(17)30092-5.pdf.

World Health Organization. 2020. "Adolescent Mental Health." Accessed February 23. www.who.int/news-room/fact-sheets/detail/adolescent-mental-health.

Zero to Three. 1994. DC 0–3: *Diagnostic Classification of Mental Health and Developmental Disorders of Infancy and Early Childhood*. www.zerotothree.org.

———. 2005. DC 0–3: *Diagnostic Classification of Mental Health and Developmental Disorders of Infancy and Early Childhood*. www.zerotothree.org.

———. 2016. *Diagnostic Classification of Mental Health and Developmental Disorders of Infancy and Early Childhood DC:0–5*. www.zerotothree.org.

INDEX

abuse and neglect of children
    extent of, 107
    risk factors for, 108–110
ACEs Aware, 179
activities
    large- and small-group, 163
    materials for, 164–166
    to support emotional wellbeing and professional boundaries, 40–42
    for transitions, 169–170
activity markers of emotional temperature, 93
adolescents
    developmental relationships and, 121
    stress and, 25–26, 118–119
    suicide, 26
adrenalin, 115
adults, responses to stress and trauma of, 118–119
adverse childhood experiences (ACEs)
    effects of, 26, 104–105
    resources, 179
    toxic stress and, 113
Ages and Stages Questionnaire (ASQ-3), 145
aggression, strength-based approach to, 157–158
Ainsworth, Mary, 84
American Academy of Pediatrics, 66
amygdala, 115, 116
anger
    increase in complexity and amount of, 15–16
    strength-based approach to, 157–158
Anti-bias Education for Young Children and Ourselves (Derman-Sparks, Edwards, and Goins), 133
Anti-Bias Leaders in Early Childhood Education, 179
anxiety disorders, 102–103
anxious behaviors, 159–160
assessment tools
    basic facts about, 145–146
    culture and, 131
    environment, 152
associate play, 20
attachment
    as continuum, 84
    importance, 10
    relationships and, 83

    secure
        described, 83, 84
        empathy, compassion and, 89
        positive sense of self and self-identity and, 70
        self-regulation and, 73–74
        signs of, 84–85
        Six Pillars and, 52, 53–54, 55
        social development and, 70
        socioemotional milestones of, 49
        of young children to parents and caregivers, 49–50
attention deficit hyperactivity disorder (ADHD), 101
attention-seeking behaviors, 159
Autism and Developmental Disabilities Monitoring Network Report (CDC), 100
autism spectrum disorder (ASD), 100

baby dolls, 165
behaviors
    anxiety disorders, 102–103
    attention deficit hyperactivity disorder, 101
    autism spectrum disorder, 100
    of children responding to trauma, 116–118
    of discouraged children, 3
    dramatic change in children's, 109–110
    in dyadic relationship, 2
    goals of, 156–157
    increase in complexity and amount of emotional, 15–16
    mood disorders, 103
    parental goals for children and, 79–80
    as reflection of unmet needs, 16, 17
    reflections for misguided, 160
    relationships and, 154
    sensory processing disorders, 102
    separating unmet needs from, 18
    serve-and-return, 43
    strength-based approaches for
        angry or aggressive, 157
        anxious or fearful, 159–160
        attention seeking, 159
        tantrums, 158
    understanding concerning behaviors
        basic facts about, 52
        questions to ask about, 53–54, 55–56
belonging, as primary goal of child, 3

bias
    anti-bias resources, 133, 179, 180
    implicit, 132–133
    learning, 132, 137
    strategies and reflections for understanding, 138
    understanding, 132–133
    unpacking, 133
        about cognitive development, 134–135
        about emotional development, 136
        about language development, 136–137
        about physical development, 134
        about social development, 135
bodily physical needs, 65
Bowlby, John, 84
brain
    activities, 114
    development of, 114–115
        ACEs and, 26
        factors affecting, 11, 19
        strategies and reflections for caregivers, 24
    emotions and, 116
    formation of mental representations, 85
    parts of, 71, 115
    receptive language and, 69
    relationships and, 11
    responses to stress and trauma, 113, 114, 116
    responsive caregiving and, 70
    simple versus complex language and, 160–161
    toxic stress and, 111, 112–113
The Brilliance of Black Boys: Cultivating School Success in the Early Grades (Wright and Counsell), 133
Bruner, Jerome, 67–68
burnout, 36, 45–46

caregivers
    attunement between children and, 42–43
    best practices, 37
    brain development and, 11
    children's needs and, 10, 12
    classroom control and, 91–92
    congruency between facial expression, tone of voice, and handling of child, 71

dyadic relationships and, 8–9, 44, 175
emotional world of, 89
factors considered when diagnosing mental health of children, 30–31
families and
 communicating with, 105, 126
 relationships with, 128
 supporting through cultural lens, 129–131
foundational skills needed by, 50
importance of strong professional boundaries, 40
listening attentively and authentically, 86–87
as mandated reporters of abuse and neglect, 109–110
needs of, 15–16
needs provided by, 10
open-ended questions and, 89–90
primary, 8–9, 10
professional boundaries
 activities to support, 40–42
 importance of strong, 40
 personal values and, 38
resiliency skills of, 119–120
resiliency skills of children and, 119, 120, 123
as role models, 70, 120, 155, 161
secure attachment to, 49–50
shared leadership of classroom and relationships with children, 91–92
social and emotional skills of, 40
strategies and reflections for
 brain development, 24
 emotional regulation, 95–96
 emotional vocabulary, 162–163
 fostering resiliency skills in children, 120, 123
 goals of children's behavior, 156–157, 160
 importance of, 36
 mental disorders of children, 106
 misguided behaviors, 160
 praise and encouragement, 156
 relationships, 24
 Six Pillars, 59
 sphere of influence, 147
 strength-based approaches, 171, 176
 support services, 147
 understanding culture and bias, 137–138
 understanding mental health of children, 33
 unpacking expectations of dominant culture, 134–137
strength-based language used by, 87, 154–156, 160–161
See also sphere of influence of caregivers

caregiver wellbeing
 activities that support, 40–42
 developing skills for, 37–38
 emotional world of, 44–46
 managing and expressing emotions, 35
 strategies and reflective practice for, 38–42, 47
 time and energy needed for, 35–36
 wellbeing of children and, 34–35
Carter, Margie, 95
Center on the Developing Child—Harvard University, 179
Center on the Social and Emotional Foundations for Early Learning (CSEFEL), 179
childhood messages, influence of, 91
children
 affirmation of positive attributes and strengths of, 150–151
 behaviors of discouraged, 3
 belonging as primary goal of, 3
 caregivers and resiliency skills of, 119
 caregiver wellbeing and wellbeing of, 34–35
 curriculum as co-construction between caregivers and, 91–92
 needs of, 10, 12
 strength-based approaches to underlying issues facing, 17, 174
children's development
 as continuum/sequence, 143
 milestones in, 31, 143–144
 relational skills, 77
 self and self-identity, 75
 self-regulation, 75–76
 social awareness, 76
Classroom Assessment Scoring System (CLASS), 146
classrooms
 assessment tools for, 145–146, 152
 based on mutual respect, 43, 44
 control of, 91–92
 cozy spaces, 167–169
 cultural awareness in, 74
 designing, for strength-based approaches, 90–92, 151–153
 developing resiliency skills in, 120, 121–122
 dysregulated, 43
 emotional temperature of, 92–94
 nurturing zones in, 94–95
 safety in, 65, 167–169
 social and emotional development and positive, 90–92
 spaces to continue play over time, 166–167
 wellbeing in, 82
closed family systems, 127, 128

Code of Ethical Conduct (NAEYC), 38
cognitive development
 emotions and, 88
 models of Bruner, 67–68
 social and emotional development and, 66–68
 stages of Piaget, 66–67
 unpacking expectations of dominant culture, 134–135
compassion, development of, 89
compassion fatigue, 46
connections. *See* relationships
cooperative play, 20
cortisol, 115–116
Counsell, Shelly, 133
cultural awareness and respect, as developmental competency, 76, 78–79
The Cultural Nature of Human Development (Rogoff), 129
culture
 assessment tools and, 131
 assumptions made by dominant, 132–137
 child's development and, 125
 families and
  circles of, 125
  goals for children, 79–80
  identity of, 137
  questions to ask about, 53–54, 56
  relationships, 52
 play and, 21
 role of, 58, 151
 sense of self and self-identity and, 74
 strategies and reflections for understanding, 137–138
 views of mental health, 127
curriculum
 as co-construction between caregivers and children, 91–92
 in deficit-based approaches, 131
 emotional literacy in, 164
 large- and small-group activities, 163
 play as, 18–19, 37
 transitions and routines, 169–170
Curtis, Deb, 95

deficit-based approaches
 curriculum in, 130
 described, 2
 learning in, 124–125
dental needs, 65
Derman-Sparks, Louise, 133
Designs for Living and Learning (Carter and Curtis), 95
developmentally appropriate practices (DAPs), 14
developmental relationships, 121
diagnosis
 classifications
  anxiety disorders, 102–103

186 INDEX

attention deficit hyperactivity
    disorder, 101
  autism spectrum disorder, 100
  factors in assessing, 99
  mood disorders, 103
  sensory processing disorders,
    101–102
factors considered, 30–31
importance of state-licensed
  professionals, 97, 98
making, 98–99, 103–105
Diagnostic Classification of Mental Health and Developmental Disorders of Infancy and Early Childhood DC:0-3, 29–30, 49
Diagnostic Classification of Mental Health and Developmental Disorders of Infancy and Early Childhood DC:0-5 (Zero to Three), 4, 29–30, 49, 98
disability support needs, 22–23
The Discovery Source, 179
dolls, 164–165
DSM-5 (*American Psychiatric Association: Diagnostic and Statistical Manual of Mental Disorders,* 5th edition), 29
dyadic relationships
  caregiver's contribution to, 175
  caregiver's emotional wellbeing and, 44
  classroom environments and, 43
  described, 2–3
  importance of, 8–9, 50
  nonverbal emotional cues, 86
  research and, 48–49
  serve-and-return interactions in, 43, 62, 77, 79, 86
  socioemotional milestones of, 49
  in strength-based approaches, 174
dysregulated classrooms, 43

early care and education, described, 140
Early Childhood Environment Rating Scale (ECERS-3), 146
"Early Childhood Expulsion and Bias" (First Things First Early Childhood Summit 2019), 133
Edwards, Julie Olsen, 133
emotional availability, 45
emotional development. *See* social and emotional development
emotional health
  defined, 5
  See also caregiver wellbeing
emotional labor, 35
emotional literacy
  as cornerstone of strength-based learning and development, 163
  language for expressing emotions, 88
    activities, 162, 164–166
      naming emotions, 71

nonverbal emotional cues, 86
pauses, 89
short-term positive statements, 155
in targeted strength-based approach, 160–161
unpacking expectations of dominant culture for development of, 136–137
resources for building, 161
emotional preparedness, 44
emotional skills
  basis of development of, 15
  importance of, 27
emotional temperature, 45, 92–94, 153
emotional wellbeing, defined, 5
emotions
  authentic listening and, 87
  of caregivers, 89
  connection to cognitive development, 88
  cozy spaces and, 167–169
  frontal cortex of brain and, 116
  identifying, regulating, and expressing, 88
  naming, 71, 89
  nurturing zones and, 94–95
  as overwhelming children, 17
  personal, versus professional, 38
  as physical sensations, 70–71
  reflective practice for awareness of, 89
  responsive caregiving and, 11
  scaffolding, 68–69
  understanding though emotional development, 70
  See also self-regulation
empathy, development of, 89
enactive representation model, 67
encouragement, 154, 155, 156
environment. *See* classrooms; high-quality learning environments
Environmental Rating Scale, 152
expressive language, 69

families
  Ages and Stages Questionnaire (ASQ-3) and, 145
  caregivers and
    affirming positive attributes and strengths of, 151
    communicating with, 105, 126
    relationships with, 128
    support of, through cultural lens, 129–131
  culture and
    circles of, 125
    goals for children, 79–80
    identity and, 137
    questions to ask about, 53–54, 56
    relationships, 52
  development of mental health, 58

  influence on development of children of, 9
  members of, 10
  risk factors for abuse and neglect of children, 108–109
  societal messages and, 125
  in strength-based approaches, 124, 126, 151
  systems of
    closed, 127, 128
    open, 127–128
Family Child Care Environment Rating Scale-3 (FCCERS-3), 146
fearful behaviors, 159–160
feelings. *See* emotions
free play. *See* play
friendship skills, as part of social and emotional development, 70
frontal cortex (neocortex), 115, 116

gender and autism spectrum disorder, 100
genetics and mental health and wellbeing, 27
Goins, Catherine M., 133
Greenspan, 49

Harlow, Harry, 84
Harvard University— Center on the Developing Child, 179
health conditions affecting mental health, 104
high-quality learning environments
  importance of, 13
  NAEYC standards, 14
  play in, 18
  relationships in, 83, 172
hygiene habits, 65

iconic representation model, 67
implicit bias, 132–133
imprint of stress, 113
independent play, 20
Individualized Education Plan (IEP), 142
Individualized Family Services Plan (IFSP), 142
infants
  behavioral responses to trauma, 117–118
  caregivers and needs of, 12
  developmental competencies, 75–77
  learning environments for, 153
  resources for, 180
  signs of secure attachment, 84
  types of play by, 19–20
Infant/Toddler Environment Rating Scale (ITERS-3), 146
International Classification of Diseases, 10th edition (ICD-10, WHO), 29

INDEX 187

Kachenmeister, Cherryl, 161
K-12 schools, expulsion rate in, 16

language
- brain and simple versus complex, 161
- development of
  - importance of hearing language from birth, 68
  - learning and, 68
  - sequence of, 69
  - social and emotional development and, 68–70
- for expressing emotions
  - activities, 162, 164–166
  - naming emotions, 71, 89
  - pauses, 89
  - resources, 161
  - short-term positive statements, 155
  - in targeted strength-based approach, 160–161
  - unpacking expectations of dominant culture for development of, 136–137
- long-term resiliency builders, 155–156
- nonverbal, 86, 161
- self-regulation and, 161
- using strength-based, 87, 154–156, 160–161

learning
- deficit-based model versus strength-based model, 124–125
- by doing, 67
- image-based, 67
- language and, 68
- motor and sensory exploration, 66
- through play, 67
- through trial and error, 69

learning environments. *See* classrooms; high-quality learning environments
Lillas, C., 49
limbic system, 115
listening, attentively and authentically, 86–87

mandated reporters of abuse and neglect, 109–110
materials
- for cozy spaces, 167–168
- for play, 164–166

medical needs, 65
mental health
- clinical knowledge of, young children's, 7
- community and cultural experiences and, 125
- cultural views of, 127
- defined, 5
- DSM-5 approach to, 29
- factors influencing, 7, 27–28

families and
- development of, 58
- views of, 126–127
- impact of state of, on development, 8
- mental illness compared to, 28
- physical and health conditions affecting, 104
- play and, 64–65
Mental Health America (MHA), 19
mental health disorders
- as cause of death of children, 26
- defined, 5
- impact of, 29
- importance of early diagnosis and treatment of, 29
- mental health compared to, 28
- relationships and, 103–104
- strategies and reflections for caregivers, 106
mental health practitioners, types of, 32
mental illness. *See* mental health disorders
mental representations, 67
mild stress, 111–112
mood disorders, 103
motor development
- described, 64
- muscle memory and, 67
- passive entertainment and, 65
movement markers of emotional temperature, 93
music, 153

NAEYC (National Association for the Education of Young Children)
- basic facts about, 180
- bias and cultural assumptions, 132–133
- Code of Ethical Conduct, 38
- expulsion in K-12 schools, 16
- standards for high-quality learning environments,
National Alliance on Mental Illness (NAMI), 26–27, 105, 180
National Children's Alliance, 107
Nelsen, Jane, 3
neocortex (frontal cortex), 115, 116
neuroplasticity, 115
Nimmo, John, 133
noise
- cozy and safe spaces and, 167
- level markers of emotional temperature, 93, 153
nurturing zones in classrooms, 94–95
nutritional needs, 65

onlooker play, 20
On Monday When It Rained (Kachenmeister), 161
open-ended materials, 165
open family systems, 127–128

outdoor play, 166
parallel play, 20
parent-child relationship, 49–50, 84
parents. *See* families
Parten, Mildred, 19–20
pediatric health professionals, 142
perceptional development, described, 64
Perry, Bruce, 114
persona dolls, 165
physical conditions affecting mental health, 104
physical development
- social and emotional development and, 64–66
- types of physical needs, 65
- unpacking expectations of dominant culture, 134
Piaget, Jean, 66–67
plasticity of brain, 115
play
- areas for dramatic, 70
- areas for open-ended, creative play, and exploration, 152
- benefits of, 19
- culture and, 21
- as curriculum, 18–19, 37
- elements of, to strength-based approaches, 174
- in high-quality learning environments, 18
- importance of, 18
- learning through, 67
- materials for, 164–166
- mental health and, 64–65
- outdoor, 166
- Parten's types of, 19–20
- spaces to continue, over time, 166–167
Possibilities ECE, 180
praise, 154–155, 156
prenatal care, 27–28
preoperational reasoning stage of development, 67
preschoolers
- behavioral responses to trauma of, 118
- caregivers and needs of, 12
- signs of secure attachment, 84–85
- social and emotional competencies in
  - cultural awareness and respect, 78–79
  - relational skills, 79
  - self and self-identity, 77–78
  - self-regulation, 78
  - social awareness, 78
- types of play by, 20
primary caregivers. *See* caregivers
problem-solving skills
- early development, 67
- play and, 19

professionals
  caregiver's sphere of influence and, 140–141
  importance of state-licensed, for diagnosis, 97, 98
  pediatric health, 142
prosocial values, 14
psychiatric disorders. *See* mental health disorders
puppets, 164–165

rage, increase in complexity and amount of, 15–16
Ramsey, Patricia G., 133
receptive language, 69
reflective practice
  awareness of emotions and, 89
  elements of, 38
  emotional health of caregivers, 38–40, 40–42, 47
  emotional regulation and, 95–96
  emotional vocabulary, 162–163
  forms for and stages of, 39
  fostering resiliency skills in children, 120, 123
  goals of children's behavior, 156–157
  mental disorders of children, 106
  misguided behaviors, 160
  praise and encouragement, 156
  Six Pillars, 57–58, 59
  social and emotional development of children, 81
  strength-based approaches, 171, 176
  understanding culture and bias, 137–138
  unpacking expectations of dominant culture, 134–137
relational skills
  basic facts about, 74
  as developmental competency of infants and toddlers, 77
  as developmental competency of preschoolers, 79
relationships
  attachment and, 83
  behaviors and, 154
  developmental, 121
  formation of additional, beyond primary, 85
  guiding young children through, 15–18
  in high-quality learning environments, 83, 172
  mental health disorders and, 103–104
  secure, described, 83, 84
  sense of self and self-identity and, 73
  shared leadership of classroom and caregiver-child, 91–92
  Six Pillars and, 52, 53–54, 55

strategies and reflections for caregivers, 24
wellbeing and, 63
See also dyadic relationships
resiliency
  balance between time and energy and, 36
  basic facts about, 52
  caregivers and, of children, 119, 120, 123
  developing, 36, 119–120, 121–122
  play and, 19
  practices to enhance, 44
  questions to ask about, 53–54, 56
  reflective practice and, 38
  statements building, 155–156
resources
  ACEs, 179
  anti-bias, 133, 179, 180
  assessment tools, 145–146
  building language for expressing emotions, 161
  cultural assumptions, 133
  emotional wellness, 149
  infants, 180
  learning environments, 95
  organizations on Internet, 180
  screening tools, 145
  social and emotional development, 149, 177–178, 179
  toddlers, 180
respect
  classroom environments based on mutual, 43, 44
  as requirement of dyadic relationship, 3
responsive caregiving
  brain and, 70
  effects of, 10, 11
  as linear progression, 11
risk
  child's development and, 52
  emotional temperature of classroom and, 94
  questions to ask about, 53–54, 56
Rogoff, Barbara, 129
routines, 169, 170

safety
  elements in home, community and classroom environments and, 65, 167–169
  emotional temperature of classroom and, 94
screening tools, 145
Search Institute, 121, 180
self and self-identity
  basic facts about, 63
  defining, 72
  developing positive concept of, 63

as developmental competency of infants and toddlers, 75
as developmental competency of preschoolers, 77–78
forming, 73
secure attachments and, 70
social and culture awareness and respect, 74
wellbeing and, 63
self-care plans, 41–42
self-regulation
  basis of, 74
  in cozy spaces, 167
  as developmental competency of infants and toddlers, 75–76
  as developmental competency of preschoolers, 78
  emotional health and, 40
  language and, 161
  secure attachments and, 73–74
  strength-based approaches to, 88–89
self-sacrifice, 40
self-talk, importance of, 68
sensorimotor stage of development, 66
sensory processing disorders, 101–102
separation anxiety, 84, 85, 102
serve-and-return behaviors, 43, 62, 77, 79, 86
Siegel, Dan, 36
Six Pillars
  1. social and emotional development. *See* social and emotional development
  2. attachment and caregiving relationships. *See* attachment
  3. understanding concerning behaviors, 52, 53–54, 55–56
  4. risk and resiliency. *See* resiliency; risk
  5. family relationships and culture. *See* culture under families
  6. sphere of influence of caregivers. *See* sphere of influence of caregivers
  development of caregivers' foundational skills and, 51
  questions to ask about, 53–57
  reflections on, 57–58
  research behind, 48–50
  strategies and reflections for caregivers, 59
social and emotional development
  basic facts about, 51–52
  basis of, 62
  caregivers, reflective practice for, 82
  cognitive development and, 66–68
  emotional development, 70–71
  friendship skills and, 70
  language development and, 68–70
  physical development and, 64–66
  positive learning environments and, 90–92

INDEX

189

questions to ask, 53–55
rate of, 62–63
resources, 149, 177–178, 179
sense of self and, 63
social and emotional competencies described, 73–74
social and emotional competencies in preschoolers
  cultural awareness and respect, 78–79
  relational skills, 79
  self and self-identity, 77–78
  self-regulation, 78
  social awareness, 78
social and emotional competencies of infants and toddlers, 75–77
social development, 70
strength-based practices for scaffolding, 87–89
support needs, 22–23
unpacking expectations of dominant culture, 135–136
wellbeing and, 63, 75–79
social awareness
  as developmental competency of infants and toddlers, 76
  as developmental competency of preschoolers, 78
  sense of self and self-identity and, 74
social health, defined, 5
social skills, basis of development of, 15
socioemotional milestones, 49
solitary play, 20
sphere of influence of caregivers
  basic facts about, 52
  discovering and understanding, 139–140
  early intervention and special education partnerships, 142
  family supports, described, 141
  health and mental health partnerships, 141–142
  observing development
    milestones and, 143–144
    notes during, 144–145
  professional support and, 140–141
  questions to ask about, 53–54, 56–57
  screening and assessment within, 145–146
  strategies and reflections for caregivers, 147
storytelling patterns/arcs, 21
strength-based approaches
  affirming positive attributes and strengths of children and families, 150–151
  described, 1–2
  designing learning environments for, 90–92, 151–153
  elements of, 7–8, 174

emotional literacy and, 163
engaging children with, 129–131
families in, 124, 126, 151
language for, 87, 154–156, 160–161
learning in, 124–125
to misguided behaviors
  anger or aggression, 157–158
  anxiety, 159–160
  attention seeking, 159
  goals of, 156–157
  tantrums, 158
for scaffolding social and emotional development, 87–89
to self-regulation, 88–89
strategies and reflective practice for, 171
targeted
  1. using encouraging words, 154–156
  2. looking behind the curtain, 156–160
  3. using feeling words, 160–163
  indicators of need for, 154
trust and respect in, 3
underlying issues facing child, 17, 174
See also Six Pillars
stress
  ACEs and, 26
  adolescents and, 25–26, 118–119
  adults and, 118–119
  described, 111
  effects of caregivers experiencing, 42–43
  examples of stressors, 104–105
  measuring, 42
  mild, 111–112
  protective factors, 119–122
  responses to, 111, 113, 114, 116
  tolerable, 111, 112
  toxic, 112–113
  trauma and, 111–113
  See also adverse childhood experiences (ACEs)
suicide of adolescents, 26
support systems
  importance of, 21
  intersecting needs for, 22–23
symbolic representation model, 68

talking navigationally, 86–87
"Talking with Children about Race and Social Justice" (Nimmo), 133
tantrums, 158
Teaching Tolerance, 180
thumbprint of stress, 113
toddlers
  behavioral responses to trauma of, 118
  caregivers and needs of, 12
  developmental competencies, 75–77
  learning environments for, 153

resources for, 180
types of play by, 20
tolerable stress, 111, 112
toxic stress, 111, 112–113
transitions, 169–170
trauma
  coping strategies for, 113
  described, 111
  events causing, 112
  protective factors, 119–122
  responses to, 113–114, 116–118
  stress and, 111–113
  support needs, 22–23
trial and error learning, 69
trust, 3, 10
Turnbull, J., 49

understanding concerning behaviors
  basic facts about, 52
  questions to ask about, 53–54, 55–56
unmet needs of children
  behaviors as reflection of, 16, 17
  separating from behaviors, 18
unoccupied play, 19

values
  classroom, influencing classroom markers, 94
  demonstrating, 91
  personal versus professional, 38
Vygotsky, Lev, 68, 125

wellbeing
  community and cultural experiences and, 125
  competencies comprising, 63, 75–79
  defined, 5
  elements of, 35–36
  factors influencing, 7, 27–28
  in learning environments, 82
  resources, 149
  responsive caregiving and, 11
  trust as foundation of, 10
  See also caregiver wellbeing
What If All the Kids Are White? Anti-bias/Multicultural Education for Young Children and Families (Derman-Sparks, Ramsey, and Edwards), 133
Wieder, 49
window of tolerance, 36
World Health Organization (WHO), 26, 29
Wright, Brian L., 133

Zero to Three, 4, 29–30, 49
Zero to Three National Center for Infants, Toddlers, and Families, 180